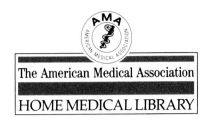

The American Medical Association

HOME MEDICAL LIBRARY

FIGHTING CANCER

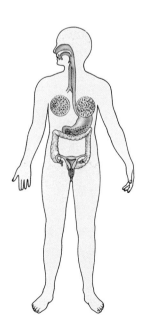

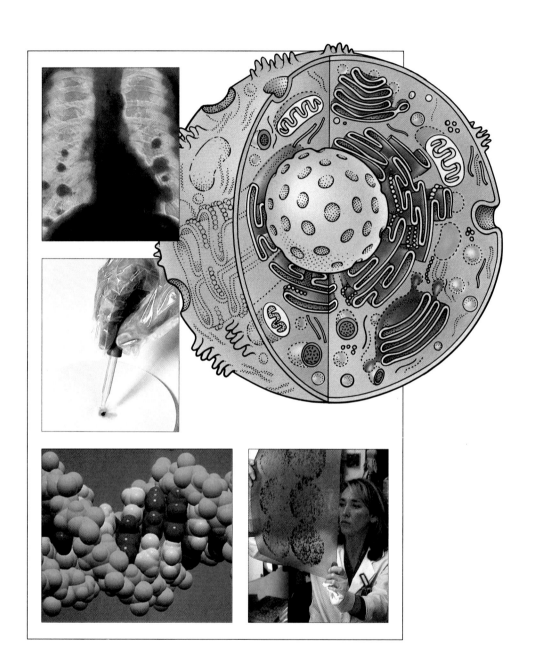

THE AMERICAN
MEDICAL ASSOCIATION

FIGHTING
CANCER

Medical Editor
CHARLES B. CLAYMAN, MD

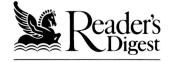

THE READER'S DIGEST ASSOCIATION, INC.
Pleasantville, New York/Montreal

Library of Congress Cataloging in Publication Data

Fighting cancer/medical editor, Charles B. Clayman.
     p.   cm. — (The American Medical Association home medical
library)
   At head of title: American Medical Association.
   Includes index.
   ISBN 0-89577-360-0
   1. Cancer — Popular works.   [1. Neoplasms — popular works.]
   I. Clayman, Charles B.   II. American Medical Association.
   III. Series.
   RC263.F483   1991   90-8503
   616.99'4 — dc20   CIP

FOREWORD

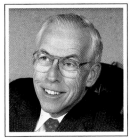

In the early 1970s, major breakthroughs in cancer treatment resulted in a dramatic improvement in the survival rates of many types of cancer – among them ovarian cancer, testicular cancer, and leukemia. To many of us, it might seem that little progress has been made in the treatment of cancer. Today, more people in developed countries are diagnosed with cancer than ever before, and the death rate of the disease is higher than it was in 1950.

Yet, paradoxically, cancer deaths have risen because we are healthier. Cancer is a disease that is more common as we age and as our life expectancy increases. Furthermore, if cancers related to tobacco are excluded, the number of deaths due to cancer has declined. Simple mortality statistics can be deceptive and mask some encouraging trends. Cure rates have improved for several types of cancer, and advances have been made in prevention and early diagnosis. If you quit smoking (or – better yet – never start), eat a varied diet, and minimize your exposure to the sun, your chances of getting cancer are cut by about half. You can improve these chances further by having the recommended cancer checkups, by regular self-examination, and by being aware of the symptoms of cancer. These measures can help you work with your doctor to catch the disease at a stage when treatment for many cancers has the greatest chance for success.

We hope this volume of the AMA Home Medical Library – which covers subjects including the causes and prevention of cancer and its diagnosis and treatment – will help you and your family better understand cancer and the ways in which doctors can now help those touched by the disease.

James S. Todd MD

JAMES S. TODD, MD
Executive Vice President
American Medical Association

CONTENTS

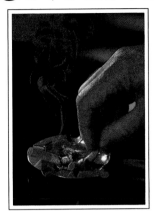

CHAPTER ONE

CANCER IN THE MODERN WORLD

INTRODUCTION

WHY DOES
CANCER OCCUR?

IS CANCER
ON THE INCREASE?

ARE WE WINNING
THE FIGHT
AGAINST CANCER?

THE GROUP OF DISEASES known as cancer has a fearsome reputation in our society. One public opinion poll confirmed that 90 percent of people dread cancer above all other threats to life, nuclear war included. Yet it is circulatory disease – the cause of heart attacks and strokes – that heads the list of common causes of death in developed countries. Cancer inspires fear because many people assume that death is the inevitable outcome once cancer has been diagnosed. The facts are less terrifying and give a firm basis for hope. True, cancer is now responsible for 20 percent of deaths in the US and about 1 million Americans are diagnosed as having cancer each year. However, of those 1 million people, 400,000 individuals will receive early and effective treatment and in time will be able to resume their

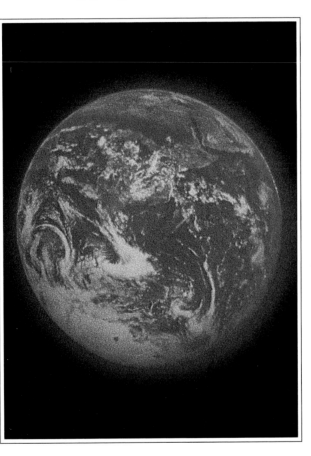

lives, many of them completely cured. Millions of dollars are invested in cancer research. As the causes of cancer become better understood, the choices we need to make to reduce our risk of acquiring the disease will become increasingly clear. In this chapter, we examine the broad picture of cancer, both in the US and worldwide. Since the 1930s, cancer in developed countries has been on the increase, an alarming trend. But it is highly significant that most of this increase is due to a steep rise in the incidence of lung cancer and that, furthermore, almost all cases of lung cancer are attributable to smoking. For many years, this largely preventable cancer has been the most common cause of cancer death in men. Now it has overtaken breast cancer as the most common cause of cancer death in women as well. The elimination of tobacco smoking, more than any other single factor, would reduce deaths from cancer, as well as reduce the incidence of other serious lung disorders such as chronic bronchitis and emphysema. Cancer affects one in three people in the US at some time in their lives. However, the prospects for these individuals are better than they have ever been. This chapter examines the techniques doctors use to beat cancer, including a range of methods for detecting cancer in its early stages (before it has spread into surrounding tissues and organs). The chances of surviving specific cancers are also examined. The fact that one out of two people with cancer now survives 5 years after treatment is remarkable evidence that the battle against cancer is not being fought in vain.

WHY DOES CANCER OCCUR?

Among the 50,000 or more separate genes in the body are 100 or so that may malfunction, making cells grow where they should not grow and producing chemicals they should not produce. These genes, known as oncogenes, are triggered by a combination of factors.

Studies linking certain areas of the world with high incidences of specific cancers have isolated suspected carcinogens (cancer-causing agents), although in some cases the way in which the carcinogen exerts its harmful effect is unknown.

Cancer of the esophagus
In northwestern France, the local apple brandy called calvados, combined with heavy smoking and a diet lacking in some vitamins and minerals, is the suspected cause of esophageal cancer.

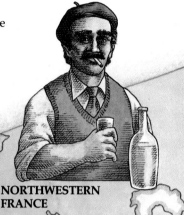

NORTHWESTERN FRANCE

Cancer of the esophagus
In certain areas of the Middle East, including Iran, there is an unexplained high incidence of esophageal cancer.

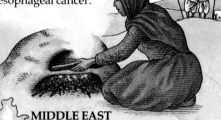

MIDDLE EAST

INDIA

Cancer of the bladder
People living near the Nile river suffer a high incidence of cancer of the bladder, caused in part by schistosomiasis, an infection with waterborne flukes found in the river.

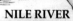

NILE RIVER

Cancer of the liver
Mozambique in southern Africa has a high incidence of cancer of the liver. A major contributing factor is infection with the hepatitis B and C viruses. Researchers have suspected a toxin produced by *Aspergillus flavus* molds growing on stored peanuts, which are an important food in the area.

CENTRAL AFRICA

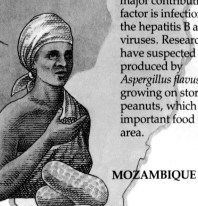

Burkitt's lymphoma
This lymphatic tissue cancer causes tumors in the jaw and abdomen; it is suspected of being caused in Africa by malaria in childhood and infection with the Epstein-Barr virus.

MOZAMBIQUE

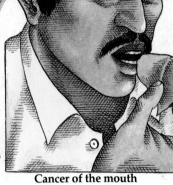

Cancer of the mouth
Cancer of the mouth is thought to be caused by smoking and chewing tobacco. The problem may be exacerbated by heavy alcohol consumption. In India, however, the practice of chewing betel leaves and nuts has led to a high incidence of cancer of the mouth. It is suspected that the betel plant contains a powerful carcinogen.

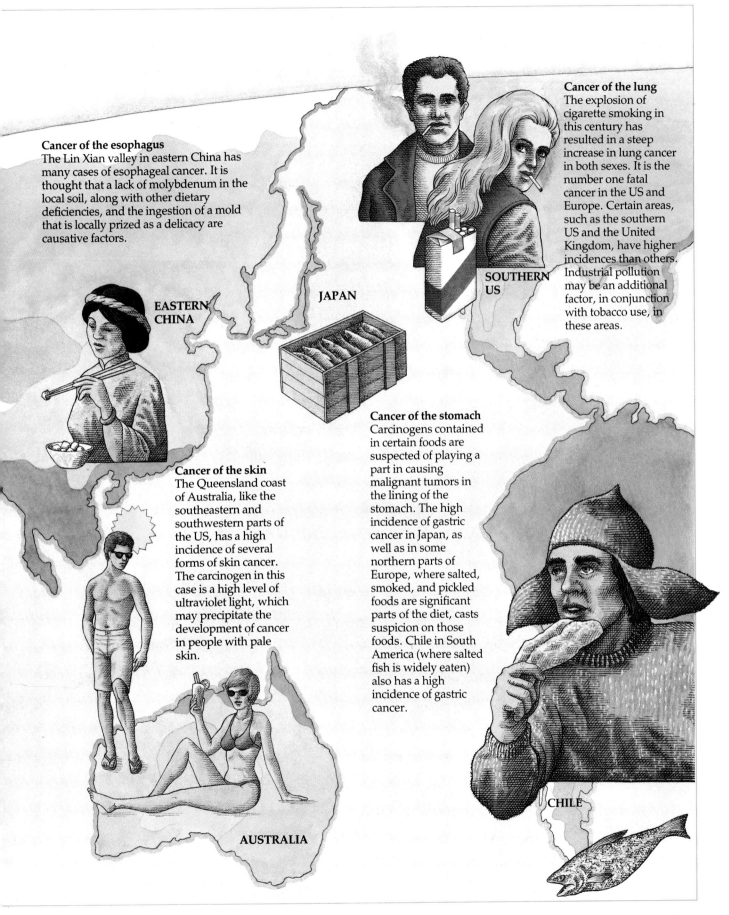

Cancer of the esophagus
The Lin Xian valley in eastern China has many cases of esophageal cancer. It is thought that a lack of molybdenum in the local soil, along with other dietary deficiencies, and the ingestion of a mold that is locally prized as a delicacy are causative factors.

Cancer of the lung
The explosion of cigarette smoking in this century has resulted in a steep increase in lung cancer in both sexes. It is the number one fatal cancer in the US and Europe. Certain areas, such as the southern US and the United Kingdom, have higher incidences than others. Industrial pollution may be an additional factor, in conjunction with tobacco use, in these areas.

EASTERN CHINA

JAPAN

SOUTHERN US

Cancer of the skin
The Queensland coast of Australia, like the southeastern and southwestern parts of the US, has a high incidence of several forms of skin cancer. The carcinogen in this case is a high level of ultraviolet light, which may precipitate the development of cancer in people with pale skin.

Cancer of the stomach
Carcinogens contained in certain foods are suspected of playing a part in causing malignant tumors in the lining of the stomach. The high incidence of gastric cancer in Japan, as well as in some northern parts of Europe, where salted, smoked, and pickled foods are significant parts of the diet, casts suspicion on those foods. Chile in South America (where salted fish is widely eaten) also has a high incidence of gastric cancer.

AUSTRALIA

CHILE

11

IS CANCER ON THE INCREASE?

Many people believe, mistakenly, that cancer is a new disease attributable in some way to the pressures and poisons of modern living. In reality, cancer has always occurred in both people and animals. Evidence of cancer has been found in the mummies of ancient Egypt and in fossilized remains of a dinosaur more than 125 million years old.

CANCER IN PERSPECTIVE

It may seem as if cancer has become much more common since the early part of this century. While it is true that there has been a rise in the death rate from the disease, the overall picture is more complex. Because people are now talking more freely about cancer, the full extent of the disease is more evident. Furthermore, people are being cured of other previously fatal diseases earlier in life. Not so long ago, many young men and women died of infections such as tuberculosis, pneumonia, and typhoid. These are now rare causes of death. Most people live to age 60 or 70, when cancer is a relatively common disease. More than one third of all people who live until 70 will eventually be found to have some form of cancer.

Greater chances of survival

About 5 million Americans alive today have been treated for cancer in the past, and about 3 million have probably been cured. Certain cancers that had a poor outlook in the past, such as acute lymphoblastic leukemia (in childhood), Hodgkin's disease, testicular cancer, choriocarcinoma of the uterus, and many cases of ovarian cancer, are now often curable. While the death rates for some cancers have not improved greatly, medicine has helped many cancer patients to live active, productive lives.

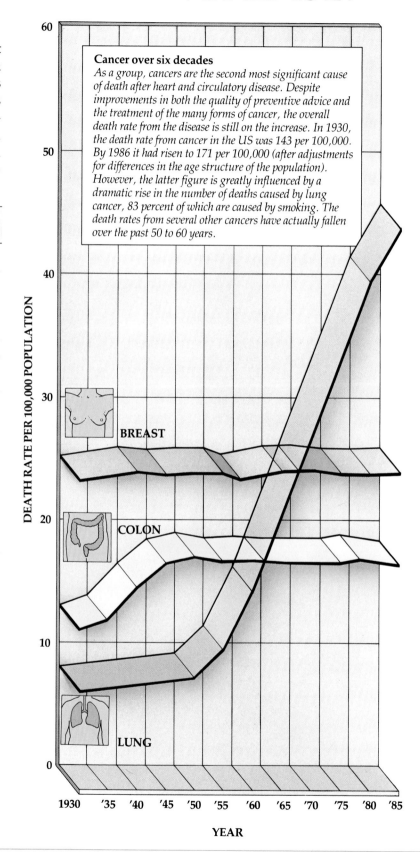

Cancer over six decades
As a group, cancers are the second most significant cause of death after heart and circulatory disease. Despite improvements in both the quality of preventive advice and the treatment of the many forms of cancer, the overall death rate from the disease is still on the increase. In 1930, the death rate from cancer in the US was 143 per 100,000. By 1986 it had risen to 171 per 100,000 (after adjustments for differences in the age structure of the population). However, the latter figure is greatly influenced by a dramatic rise in the number of deaths caused by lung cancer, 83 percent of which are caused by smoking. The death rates from several other cancers have actually fallen over the past 50 to 60 years.

DEATH RATE PER 100,000 POPULATION

BREAST

COLON

LUNG

1930 '35 '40 '45 '50 '55 '60 '65 '70 '75 '80 '85

YEAR

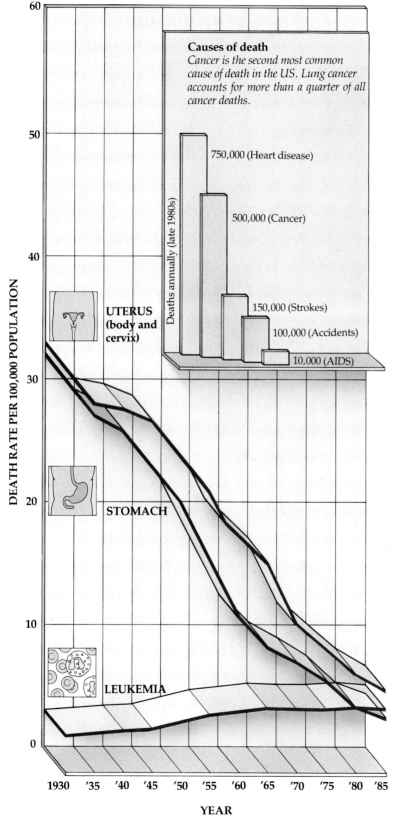

Causes of death
Cancer is the second most common cause of death in the US. Lung cancer accounts for more than a quarter of all cancer deaths.

Deaths annually (late 1980s)

750,000 (Heart disease)

500,000 (Cancer)

150,000 (Strokes)

100,000 (Accidents)

10,000 (AIDS)

DEATH RATE PER 100,000 POPULATION

UTERUS (body and cervix)

STOMACH

LEUKEMIA

YEAR

Cancer of the lung

Cancer of the lung kills more than 140,000 Americans per year, more than any other cancer. The increase in the death rate has been phenomenal. The death rate was 2.5 times greater in the early 1980s than it was in the middle 1950s.

Cancer of the breast

The death rate from cancer of the breast in women remains nearly at the same level as it was in 1930. Although lung cancer now accounts for more deaths in women than breast cancer (being fatal in 87 percent of the cases), breast cancer is more common. In Japan, breast cancer is less common than it is in the US. Earlier detection achieved through mammography should improve survival rates.

Cancer of the colon

Cancer of the colon affects about 110,000 Americans annually; half of these patients are cured completely. Although the number of diagnosed cases of cancer of the colon has risen as more people in the US reach old age, the age-adjusted death rate has varied little since 1945. A low-fiber, high-fat diet is believed to increase the risk of this cancer.

Cancer of the uterus

The death rate from cancer of the uterus, including cancer of the cervix, has dropped by more than 70 percent since the 1930s, a dramatic illustration of what can be achieved by mass screening techniques and by early detection and treatment.

Cancer of the stomach

Once a major cancer in the US, cancer of the stomach now accounts for less than 3 percent of all diagnosed cancers. The drop in the death rate from gastric cancer in the US is thought in part to be a result of the effect of refrigeration on food preservation and on changes in the ingestion of certain foods, such as pickled vegetables and smoked and salted fish.

Leukemia

The incidence of leukemia has been slowly rising in the US, but the death rate has gradually been falling for some years. There are four main types of leukemia. Acute lymphoblastic leukemia is the most common of the childhood cancers.

ARE WE WINNING THE FIGHT AGAINST CANCER?

Central to the campaign against all forms of cancer is a thorough and detailed understanding of the disease. In recent years, researchers in the field of molecular biology have discovered a wealth of new information concerning the behavior of both healthy and cancerous cells at the most basic chemical and genetic level. The influence of carcinogenic factors such as chemicals, viruses, and radiation on genetic material, especially in people who have a known genetic predisposition, is also under rigorous investigation. Building on the results of this research, it has been possible to develop a new generation of anticancer procedures and treatments.

MRI and cancer
Magnetic resonance imaging (MRI) is a technique that uses the magnetic properties of the atom to produce cross-sectional images of the body. MRI is valuable in confirming a diagnosis of cancer and can detect brain tumors otherwise concealed by bone. A tumor appears in a scan as a change in normal anatomy; the abnormality can then be enhanced by computer. The scan at right shows a cross section through the brain at the level of the eyes.

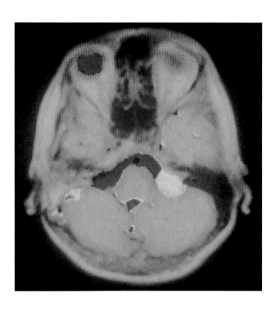

Radiation therapy
Radiation is used to treat a variety of cancers directly and to destroy cancer cells that still remain after surgery or other treatments have been carried out. Ionizing radiation, in the form of X-rays, is sent through the diseased tissue, destroying or slowing the development of abnormal cells.

Generator produces beam of radiation

Beam is focused on tumor

The healing beam
This patient with a skin cancer (shown right) underwent radiation therapy. Healthy tissue was soon reclaiming the former site of the tumor (far right).

EARLY DETECTION AND EFFECTIVE TREATMENT

Doctors cannot overemphasize the importance of early detection of all cancers. For example, the incidence of invasive (spreading) cervical cancer has been dropping for more than 30 years. This can be attributed to mass screening involving the cervical smear (Pap) test, which was first introduced in the 1940s. The Pap test allows discovery of the cancer at earlier, localized stages, permitting treatments that are curative. There has also been phenomenal development in the technology that allows doctors to see images of cancer in the body (without surgery). These images play a vital part in detecting tumors before they invade surrounding tissue and become increasingly difficult for doctors to treat.

Improving therapy

The established methods of treating cancers are chemotherapy, radiation therapy, surgery, and hormonal treatment.

In some cases, multiple techniques are used in sequence to treat a cancer.

In chemotherapy, anticancer drugs are injected into the body or taken orally to kill cancer cells or to prevent their multiplication. These drugs also have a harmful effect on healthy cells and cause severe side effects, but advances have enabled drugs to be "tailored" to latch onto specific types of cancer cells with less damage to the surrounding tissue (see TARGETING TUMORS, at right).

Radiation therapy harnesses the effects of ionizing radiation to kill the multiplying cancerous cells of a tumor. This treatment, too, has been associated with damage to surrounding tissue. However, in many cases it is now possible to target the radiation primarily onto the tumor site. Targeting of both drugs and radiation onto a tumor site minimizes the side effects of these treatments for the patient.

TARGETING TUMORS

Antibodies – substances made by the body's immune system – can now be mass-produced in a laboratory. When injected into the body, some of these monoclonal antibodies bind to antigens (markers) on the surface of cancer cells. By attaching an anticancer drug to a monoclonal antibody, the drug can be "targeted" to a tumor. The drug then kills only the abnormal cells. The drug that is attached to the monoclonal antibody can be injected only once, however. After that, antibodies to the antibody are formed.

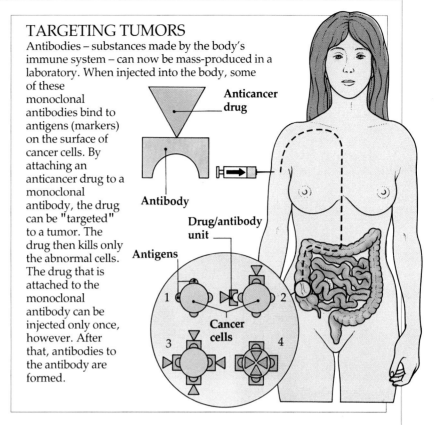

BONE MARROW TRANSPLANTATION

Very high doses of radiation and chemotherapy, which would otherwise be fatal, may be used to treat certain cancers, thanks to techniques that replace destroyed bone marrow with healthy donor marrow. A sibling or another person having identical major genetic markers may be the donor (allogeneic transplantation). Today there are registries of thousands of possible donors whose marrow can be used if it can be matched identically or almost identically to the patient. There is about a one in four chance that a sibling will be a suitable donor and, currently, only a one in 20,000 chance of finding a donor through a registry. For certain cancers, the patient is his or her own donor (autologous transplantation), providing there are no cancer cells in the bone marrow.

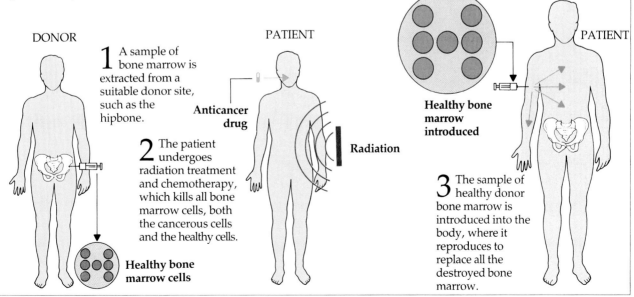

DONOR

1 A sample of bone marrow is extracted from a suitable donor site, such as the hipbone.

Healthy bone marrow cells

PATIENT

Anticancer drug

2 The patient undergoes radiation treatment and chemotherapy, which kills all bone marrow cells, both the cancerous cells and the healthy cells.

Radiation

Healthy bone marrow introduced

PATIENT

3 The sample of healthy donor bone marrow is introduced into the body, where it reproduces to replace all the destroyed bone marrow.

THE OUTLOOK FOR CANCER

People's awareness of potentially harmful environmental factors is highly significant in preventing cancer. Strong sunlight, tobacco smoke, excess alcohol, nuclear radiation, and exposure to such substances as asbestos, chromium, nickel, and polyvinyl chloride are factors over which individuals, or society as a whole, have some degree of control.

Screening

Knowledge of the disease is also important. Breast and testicular self-examination and regular screening procedures such as the cervical smear (Pap) test and mammography are essential if growing cancers are to be detected when they are small enough for possible cure. In addition, everyone should know the early symptoms that may signal cancer.

The outlook for certain cancers has improved greatly over the past 30 years. For example, in the early 1960s only 4 percent of children with acute lymphoblastic leukemia survived for 5 years. Of those who were diagnosed with acute lymphoblastic leukemia in the early 1980s, 68 percent survived for 5 years and virtually all were cured. In some cancer centers, 75 percent of these children survive for 5 years. Drug treatments, radiation therapy, and bone marrow transplants have all contributed to this improvement.

The treatments for Hodgkin's disease and testicular cancer have been similarly successful and people who have these diseases can now often be completely cured. Research continues into new therapies for other forms of cancer, such as chronic myeloid leukemia.

CANCER WATCH

See your doctor immediately if you have any of the following symptoms.

◆ Change in bowel or bladder habit
◆ A sore that does not heal
◆ Unusual bleeding or discharge
◆ Thickening or lump in a breast or elsewhere
◆ Indigestion or difficulty swallowing
◆ Obvious change in a wart or mole
◆ Chronic cough or hoarseness

HOW MANY PEOPLE SURVIVE AFTER A CANCER DIAGNOSIS?

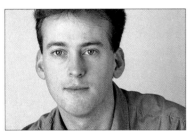

Testicular cancer
Eight years ago, Ian (above) had a lump in one testicle. It was diagnosed as a malignant tumor and the testicle was removed. He has had no recurrence.

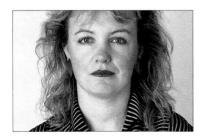

Hodgkin's disease
Helen (above) had the lymphatic cancer Hodgkin's disease, but was cured by radiation therapy and drugs.

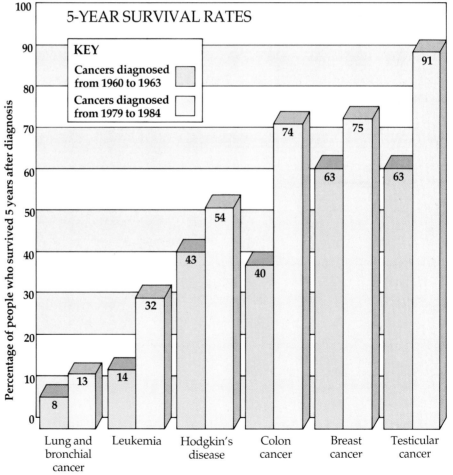

5-YEAR SURVIVAL RATES

KEY
Cancers diagnosed from 1960 to 1963
Cancers diagnosed from 1979 to 1984

Percentage of people who survived 5 years after diagnosis

Lung and bronchial cancer	Leukemia	Hodgkin's disease	Colon cancer	Breast cancer	Testicular cancer
8 / 13	14 / 32	43 / 54	40 / 74	63 / 75	63 / 91

CASE HISTORY
A CURABLE CANCER

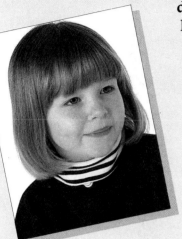

I**N THE PAST MONTH** Susan has been sick a couple of times with a sore throat. Two days ago another sore throat developed. Susan feels terrible, looks pale, and has no appetite. Her mother decides to take Susan to see the pediatrician because there has been no sign of improvement in her daughter's condition.

PERSONAL DETAILS
Name Susan Cooper
Age 6
Occupation Student
Family Father and mother are both in good health.

MEDICAL BACKGROUND
Other than chickenpox and a middle-ear infection, Susan has had no significant diseases or disorders.

THE CONSULTATION
Susan has a temperature of 100°F, swollen glands in her neck, and an enlarged spleen. She also has some spots on her arms and legs, which are due to tiny areas of bleeding into her skin. The pediatrician takes a specimen of blood, which reveals a low level of oxygen-carrying red cells and a raised number of white cells, mostly the type known as lymphocytes. He suggests that Susan go into a hospital for more tests as quickly as possible.

THE DIAGNOSIS
At the hospital a specimen of bone marrow is taken from Susan's hipbone. The laboratory examination shows that her bone marrow is full of abnormal, immature, white cells (leukemic cells) that are interfering with production of normal blood cells (red cells, white cells, and platelets). She has ACUTE LYMPHOBLASTIC

LEUKEMIA. Susan's blood is deficient in red cells, which is making her anemic; the low level of normal white cells is making her susceptible to infections, such as the sore throat, and the deficiency in platelets is causing the bleeding into her skin.

THE TREATMENT
Susan is given drugs that will kill the cancer cells in her bone marrow. At the same time, these drugs damage the healthy cells in the bone marrow. This means that, at first, Susan becomes even more anemic and needs repeated blood transfusions. She also must have drugs injected into her spinal fluid and a course of radiation therapy to destroy any leukemic cells.

Susan stays in the hospital in a special isolation room designed to reduce the risk of her being exposed to bacteria and viruses.

THE OUTCOME
After about 6 weeks, blood tests reveal that the leukemic cells have disappeared, and the leukemia is said to have entered a period of remission. Susan is allowed to go home, although she will need more drug treatment and blood tests at regular intervals. Five years later, Susan is still well and probably cured.

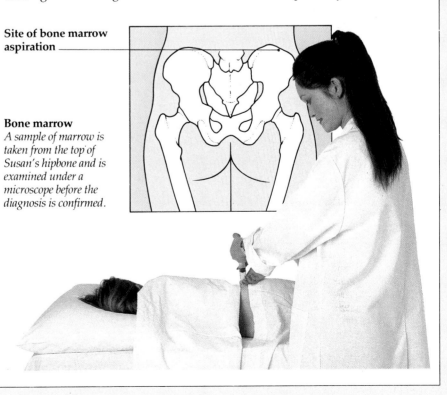

Site of bone marrow aspiration

Bone marrow
A sample of marrow is taken from the top of Susan's hipbone and is examined under a microscope before the diagnosis is confirmed.

CHAPTER TWO

WHAT IS CANCER?

INTRODUCTION

UNDERSTANDING THE NATURE OF CANCER

THE EFFECTS OF CANCER

THE WORD "CANCER" is one of the few layperson's terms universally accepted and used by the medical profession. One misconception about the term is that it describes a single disease. In fact, the word cancer is used because it is applicable to at least 200 apparently different conditions. Cancer can involve virtually any tissue or organ of the body. It can strike one or two organs initially or show up as a secondary invader from elsewhere in the body. Cancer may take many diverse forms, varying widely in their significance for health and life. Some cancers are so minor that they can be cured by a needle prick and 10 minutes of painless surgery. Others are so significant that long before any symptoms appear, the disease may already be beyond a cure. The common cancer of the airways in the lungs caused by cigarette smoking is often of this type.

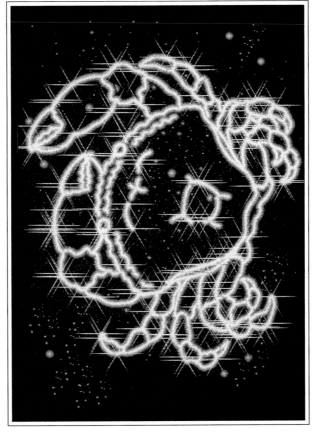

In spite of the variation among individual cancers, there is an important sense in which cancer is a single disease. All cancers consist of abnormal cells that show the characteristic of unrestrained growth; there is evidence that this characteristic can be the result of changes in a cell's genetic material (the DNA), which controls growth. In the first section of this chapter, UNDERSTANDING THE NATURE OF CANCER, we examine what has been discovered about the biology of cancer and review the areas of the body most commonly affected. The behavior of healthy cells is compared with the behavior of cancerous cells to illustrate the uncontrolled growth and disruption of specialized cell function that is characteristic of cancers. The development of cancer is traced – from the mutation of normal cells to the formation of a cancerous tumor and its potential spread into other parts of the body via the lymphatic system or the bloodstream.

Cancer can have a wide range of effects on the body. In THE EFFECTS OF CANCER, we describe some of the symptoms cancers produce. Certain types of cancer lead to vague, nonspecific symptoms that may at first be attributed to a less alarming cause. Some cancers produce no symptoms until they are at an advanced stage. Others produce worrisome effects close to the site of the cancer. Although many cancers develop without warning, there are certain signs that are typical of specific cancers. The case history on breast cancer demonstrates the dangers of ignoring such warning signs and thus reducing the chances of effective treatment.

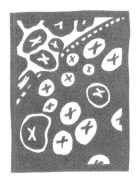

UNDERSTANDING THE NATURE OF CANCER

Cancer is a disease that causes cells to grow when they should not and to migrate to tissues where they should not be. The cells of the body normally operate in "communities" that display rigorously regulated growth; each cell has a special function. In all cancers, whatever their cause, the normal restraints on growth are lost and cells no longer function as they should.

The basis of all cancers lies in a series of biological events that leads to abnormal cell behavior. To understand what goes wrong, researchers have been working to increase their knowledge of the normal functioning of body cells.

CELL BEHAVIOR

Not all cells are alike but they have so many features in common that one can speak in terms of a "typical" cell.

CONTROL OF TISSUE GROWTH

Healthy cells in the body operate in groups that send signals from cell to cell. These signals help to regulate growth. In cancer, the cells fail to produce these signals or to respond to them.

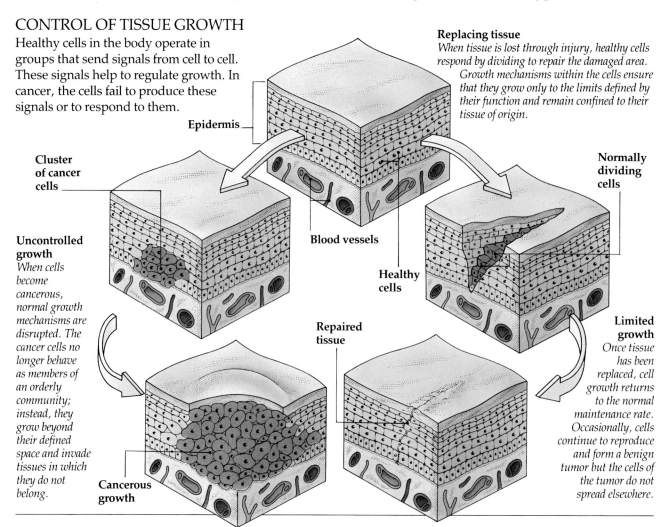

Epidermis

Replacing tissue
When tissue is lost through injury, healthy cells respond by dividing to repair the damaged area. Growth mechanisms within the cells ensure that they grow only to the limits defined by their function and remain confined to their tissue of origin.

Cluster of cancer cells

Uncontrolled growth
When cells become cancerous, normal growth mechanisms are disrupted. The cancer cells no longer behave as members of an orderly community; instead, they grow beyond their defined space and invade tissues in which they do not belong.

Blood vessels

Normally dividing cells

Healthy cells

Repaired tissue

Cancerous growth

Limited growth
Once tissue has been replaced, cell growth returns to the normal maintenance rate. Occasionally, cells continue to reproduce and form a benign tumor but the cells of the tumor do not spread elsewhere.

The healthy cell

Cells in the lining of the intestines, the deep layers of the skin, and the bone marrow divide rapidly and continuously. Cells in the muscles divide much more slowly. Those in the brain hardly divide at all. The way in which cell production is controlled is still not fully understood. One certain factor is the ability of the cells to inhibit each other's growth once they come into contact with each other. This property, known as contact inhibition, ensures that cells grow only to the limits of their defined space and then stop. Thus, when cells are tightly packed together, they reproduce slowly. If the cell density is reduced, cell reproduction is increased. Liver cells normally grow very slowly. However, if a piece of liver is removed, the surrounding cells will multiply rapidly until the deficiency in tissue is restored. This may occur, in part, because the cells secrete growth factors that act on neighboring cells and on themselves. However, when the cells become tightly packed again, secretion of the growth factors ceases.

The wayward cell

Cancer is thought to develop from a single cell or from a small pool of cells after changes have occurred in their DNA – the genetic material carrying the coded information that instructs the cells how to behave. A few cancers occur as a result of an inherited genetic abnormality but most are caused by environmental agents that are capable of causing genetic mutations. Anything capable of changing genetic material is called a carcinogen. We still have much to learn about the factors that result in the production of cancers (carcinogenesis). However, scientists have identified three types of carcinogenic agents – certain chemicals, radiation, and viruses. These agents and carcinogenesis are addressed in Chapter Three, CAUSES AND PREVENTION.

THE RATE OF TUMOR ENLARGEMENT

A cancer that begins with one small group of cells must divide about 25 to 30 times (provided there is a low rate of cell death) before it reaches a mass large enough to be detected by techniques such as X-rays, scans, or endoscopy. The smallest such mass is about 1 gram. A tumor, such as the one shown below, may take 5 years to reach a detectable size by doubling its mass at a rate of six times a year. However, in most tumors there is a high rate of cell death, so it can take many more years to grow to this size.

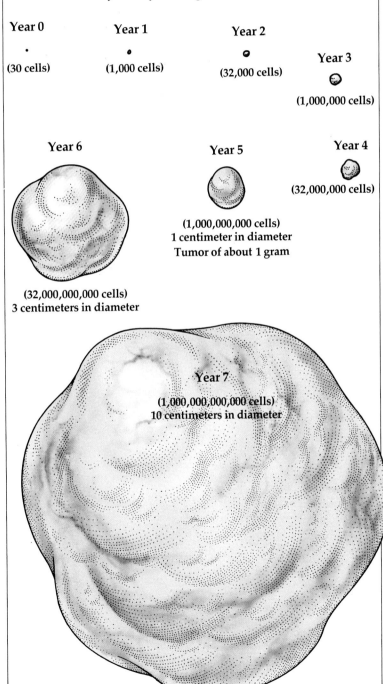

Year 0

(30 cells)

Year 1

(1,000 cells)

Year 2

(32,000 cells)

Year 3

(1,000,000 cells)

Year 4

(32,000,000 cells)

Year 5

(1,000,000,000 cells)
1 centimeter in diameter
Tumor of about 1 gram

Year 6

(32,000,000,000 cells)
3 centimeters in diameter

Year 7

(1,000,000,000,000 cells)
10 centimeters in diameter

WHERE DOES CANCER STRIKE?

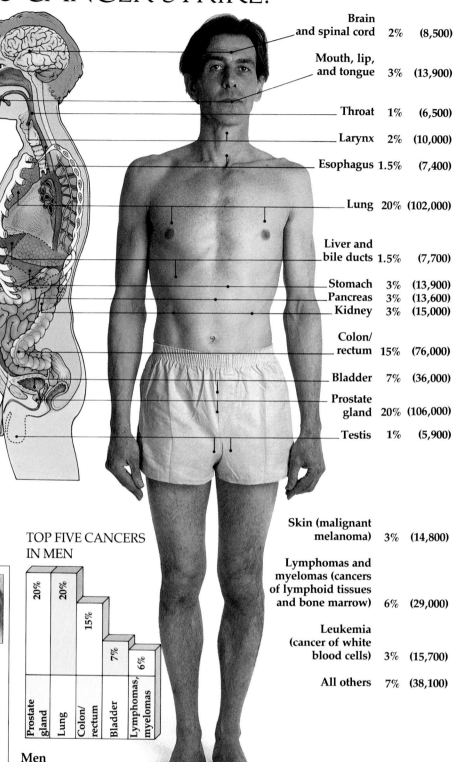

MEN

The charts on these two pages show the common sites for cancer occurrence in American men, women, and children. For each cancer, the figure expressed is a percentage of the total cancers that occur in these groups, excluding non-melanoma skin cancers (see box on SKIN CANCERS, below). The numbers in parentheses refer to estimated cases in 1990. Although cancer can originate in any part of the body, about three quarters of all cancers originate in nine or ten major sites. Apart from the skin, these sites are the lung, the colon/rectum, pancreas, and the lymphatic and blood-forming tissues in both sexes; the prostate gland and bladder in men; and the breast and uterus (including the cervix) in women. Some cancers obviously occur only in men or in women. However, even among cancers affecting both sexes, there are differences in incidence. For example, blad-der cancer is much more com-mon in men and thyroid cancer is more common in women.

Brain and spinal cord	2%	(8,500)
Mouth, lip, and tongue	3%	(13,900)
Throat	1%	(6,500)
Larynx	2%	(10,000)
Esophagus	1.5%	(7,400)
Lung	20%	(102,000)
Liver and bile ducts	1.5%	(7,700)
Stomach	3%	(13,900)
Pancreas	3%	(13,600)
Kidney	3%	(15,000)
Colon/rectum	15%	(76,000)
Bladder	7%	(36,000)
Prostate gland	20%	(106,000)
Testis	1%	(5,900)
Skin (malignant melanoma)	3%	(14,800)
Lymphomas and myelomas (cancers of lymphoid tissues and bone marrow)	6%	(29,000)
Leukemia (cancer of white blood cells)	3%	(15,700)
All others	7%	(38,100)

SKIN CANCERS

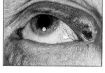

Nonmelanoma skin cancer, such as that shown at right, has been omitted from these charts partly because it is so successfully treated and partly because no accurate records of its incidence are maintained. However, it is estimated that more than 600,000 cases of nonmelanoma skin cancer occur annually in the US.

TOP FIVE CANCERS IN MEN

Prostate gland	Lung	Colon/rectum	Bladder	Lymphomas, myelomas
20%	20%	15%	7%	6%

Men

Cancers of the prostate, lung, and colon/rectum are the most common in men. About one in four men will have one of these cancers if he lives long enough. Among men in their 20s and 30s, testicular cancer is the most common type. Malignant melanoma is also increasing in incidence.

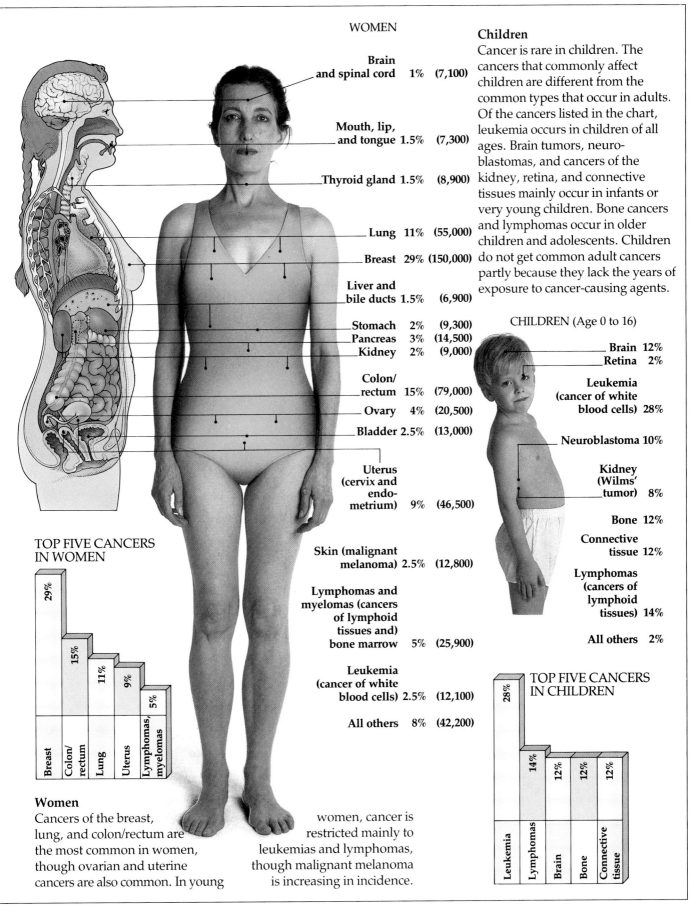

WOMEN

Brain and spinal cord	1%	(7,100)
Mouth, lip, and tongue	1.5%	(7,300)
Thyroid gland	1.5%	(8,900)
Lung	11%	(55,000)
Breast	29%	(150,000)
Liver and bile ducts	1.5%	(6,900)
Stomach	2%	(9,300)
Pancreas	3%	(14,500)
Kidney	2%	(9,000)
Colon/rectum	15%	(79,000)
Ovary	4%	(20,500)
Bladder	2.5%	(13,000)
Uterus (cervix and endometrium)	9%	(46,500)
Skin (malignant melanoma)	2.5%	(12,800)
Lymphomas and myelomas (cancers of lymphoid tissues and) bone marrow	5%	(25,900)
Leukemia (cancer of white blood cells)	2.5%	(12,100)
All others	8%	(42,200)

Children

Cancer is rare in children. The cancers that commonly affect children are different from the common types that occur in adults. Of the cancers listed in the chart, leukemia occurs in children of all ages. Brain tumors, neuroblastomas, and cancers of the kidney, retina, and connective tissues mainly occur in infants or very young children. Bone cancers and lymphomas occur in older children and adolescents. Children do not get common adult cancers partly because they lack the years of exposure to cancer-causing agents.

CHILDREN (Age 0 to 16)

Brain	12%
Retina	2%
Leukemia (cancer of white blood cells)	28%
Neuroblastoma	10%
Kidney (Wilms' tumor)	8%
Bone	12%
Connective tissue	12%
Lymphomas (cancers of lymphoid tissues)	14%
All others	2%

TOP FIVE CANCERS IN WOMEN

- Breast 29%
- Colon/rectum 15%
- Lung 11%
- Uterus 9%
- Lymphomas, myelomas 5%

TOP FIVE CANCERS IN CHILDREN

- Leukemia 28%
- Lymphomas 14%
- Brain 12%
- Bone 12%
- Connective tissue 12%

Women

Cancers of the breast, lung, and colon/rectum are the most common in women, though ovarian and uterine cancers are also common. In young women, cancer is restricted mainly to leukemias and lymphomas, though malignant melanoma is increasing in incidence.

Tumor growth
A benign tumor may grow very large and damage surrounding structures by compressing them, but the cells of the tumor do not invade other organs. By contrast, the cells of a cancerous tumor can invade surrounding tissues and organs or spread to other parts of the body. These differences are illustrated below by comparing the possible growth of a benign tumor and a malignant tumor of the colon.

DIFFERENT TYPES OF TUMORS

All solid cancers are tumors, but not all tumors are cancers. The word "tumor" is a Latin word meaning swelling and was originally used to describe any kind of swelling. Today it is used to describe both benign (noncancerous) tumors and malignant (cancerous) tumors.

What are benign tumors?

Benign tumors are not cancers. They are simply clumps of cells that, while still closely resembling the tissue from which they have arisen, have begun to reproduce and multiply faster than they should. Warts and moles are familiar examples. Such tumors often develop a strong fibrous shell or capsule around themselves. The cells of a benign tumor never invade other tissues or spread to other parts of the body, as do the cells of malignant tumors.

In general, benign tumors do not seriously damage the body. However, if they grow very large, they may cause extensive damage by exerting pressure on surrounding structures. Most benign tumors require no treatment; those that do can be removed. Occasionally, however, a change occurs in the cells of a benign tumor that causes it to become cancerous.

Benign tumors can affect almost all tissues. The majority of tumors of the breast are benign, as are the majority of tumors of the body of the uterus. A large number of skin tumors are benign. Many tumors that involve the brain are benign. However, because the brain is enclosed in a rigid bone casing, anything growing inside may cause damage by pressing on the internal brain structures. As a result, benign tumors of the brain and of the membranes covering the brain (the meninges) are always dangerous.

Malignant tumors

The features of malignant tumors are different from those of benign tumors. Malignant tumor cells do not remain in a well-defined, circumscribed lump. Rather, they invade surrounding tissues and may stretch out, much like the claws of a crab (from which the term cancer is derived). Cancers burrow into adjacent tissues and organs, become incorporated into them, and often destroy them. Malignant tumor cells also spread along tissue surfaces and spread into blood and lymph vessels to invade organs elsewhere in the body.

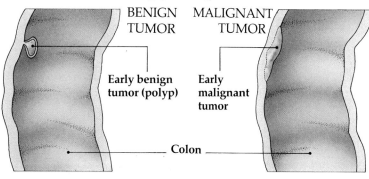

BENIGN TUMOR   MALIGNANT TUMOR

Early benign tumor (polyp)

Early malignant tumor

Colon

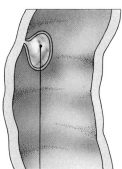

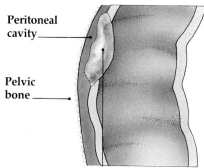

Peritoneal cavity

Pelvic bone

Benign tumor growing by expansion only

Malignant tumor has invaded the wall of the colon and peritoneal surface

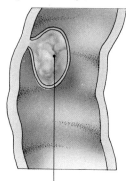

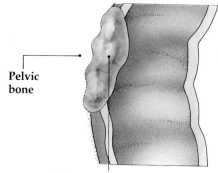

Pelvic bone

Further growth; no spread

The spreading tumor has become attached to the pelvic bone

UNDERSTANDING CANCER CLASSIFICATIONS

The many different types of cancer are given individual names that almost always include the name of the tissue or organ from which they originate. In addition to this classification, all cancers may be divided into three main groups, which are described below according to their tissue of origin.

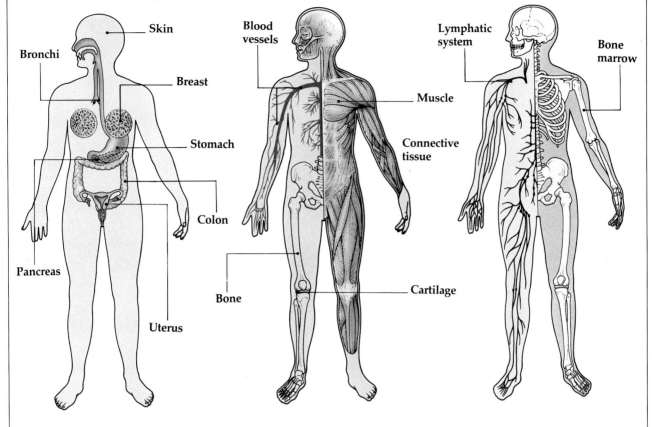

Group 1: Carcinomas
Carcinomas are the most common group of cancers. They arise from cells in the surfaces lining any part of the body. Carcinomas include cancers arising in the bronchi (lung cancers), breast cancer, skin cancer, and cancers of the stomach, pancreas, colon, and uterus.

Group 2: Sarcomas
Sarcomas arise from the substance of the body's supporting and connective tissues, such as muscles, tendons, and bones. Sarcomas are less common than carcinomas, but there are more different types of sarcomas than there are types of carcinomas.

Group 3: Other types
A third class of cancers, today usually considered distinct from the sarcomas, are those originating in the bone marrow or lymphatic systems. These include the leukemias, lymphomas, and myelomas.

THE SPREAD OF CANCER

A cancer that lies at the site where it originally developed is called a primary tumor. The borders of an invasive primary tumor are often unclear, and it may be difficult to determine how far the tumor has spread. This is why surgeons, when possible, remove a considerable zone of apparently normal tissue surrounding the tumor.

The problem of metastasis

The complete removal of a cancer often fails to prevent a recurrence at the original site, in nearby structures, or in other parts of the body. This is because cancer cells often spread from the primary tumor through the lymphatic system or bloodstream before treatment is started. This process is called metastasis.

During metastasis, a primary tumor sends microscopically small, inapparent, secondary colonies to other sites in

COMMON CANCER TERMINOLOGY

Cancer A general term for about 200 diseases in which there is uncontrolled cell growth
Carcinomas Cancers arising from surface membranes
Leukemias Cancers of white blood cells in the bone marrow
Lymphomas Cancers of the lymphoid tissues
Myelomas Cancers of plasma cells in the bone marrow
Oncology The study of benign and malignant tumors
Sarcomas Cancers arising from muscle, supporting tissues, and connective tissues

the body. In such cases, the removal of a primary tumor does not cure the cancer, since the secondary colonies will eventually form tumors. Chemotherapy, which acts throughout the body, is often used (in addition to surgery) when such metastases are suspected.

The lymphatic system is easily invaded by cancer cells. Tumor cells that enter the lymph vessels are usually held for a time in the lymph glands into which the vessels drain. Enlargement of the nearby lymph glands is often the first sign of a cancer. Surgeons usually try to remove lymph glands close to the site of a tumor so that no malignant cells are left behind.

In addition to local spread and metastasis, cancers can grow into body cavities and onto free surfaces such as the peritoneum (which lines the abdomen) or the pleura (which lines the lung). In such cases, the tumor derives nourishment from the fluid secreted by the surface

membranes and, as a result, spreads from the initial growth. Tumors in such areas often produce fluid themselves, which provides yet another vehicle for the cancer to spread. This often occurs in lung or ovarian cancer and leads to the formation of multiple small tumors and a collection of fluid in the abdomen (ascites) or chest (effusion).

The body's reaction

The body is not defenseless against the development and spread of cancers. The body's immune system fights cancer cells in a manner similar to that by which it fights infection. It is probable that once we reach middle age, cancer cells have already arisen several times in our bodies but have been destroyed by an efficient immune system. People whose immune systems have been weakened, such as those who have AIDS, are more susceptible to certain types of cancer.

Examining cancer tissue
By examining a thin slice of tissue under a microscope, a pathologist can identify malignant cells. The two photographs at right show cells taken from the lining of the cervix. The cells in the bottom slide show evidence of malignancy because they have abnormally large, dark nuclei. In the normal tissue sample shown in the top slide, each cell has a large area of cytoplasm and a small, centrally placed nucleus.

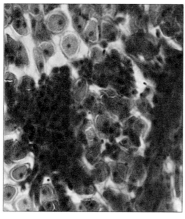

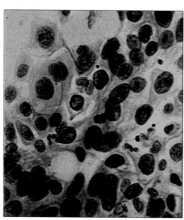

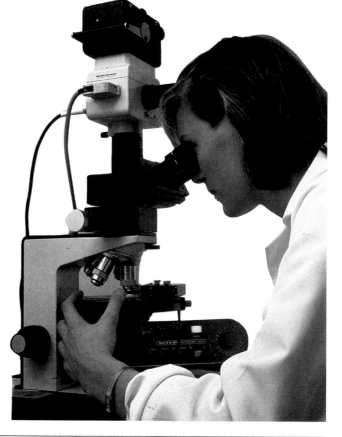

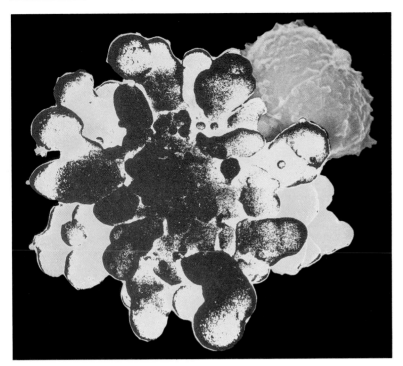

DEGREES OF MALIGNANCY

A pathologist can often tell by examining cancer tissue under a microscope whether the cancer is fast or slow growing. A fast-growing cancer that invades the tissues around it is said to be highly malignant. The degree of malignancy assessed in this way is often called the tumor grade. Some tumors closely resemble the parent tissue and are not greatly different in structure. These cancers are said to be differentiated. Other cancers are called "primitive" or undifferentiated. They are tumors that have little or no capacity to form recognizable tissues. Their cells are often larger than normal and their nuclear structure is abnormal. Although highly malignant tumors are often made up of primitive cells, well-differentiated cells may have the same tendency to spread.

The differences between healthy cells and cancer cells also make it possible for a skilled pathologist, using a microscope, to examine cells taken from the skin and a variety of body fluids and internal surfaces to look for those that might suggest malignancy.

How the body attacks cancerous cells
Once antigens (protein markers) have formed on the surface of cancer cells, the immune system can recognize them as foreign bodies and send white blood cells (lymphocytes) to attack them. The color-enhanced photograph above shows this process taking place. The green cell, a T-lymphocyte killer cell, has attached itself to the surface of a large cancerous tumor cell. The lymphocyte must make contact with the cancer cell to destroy it. In this case, the cancer cell is likely to survive because it has formed a protective barrier of blisters to prevent complete contact with the T-lymphocyte.

HOW CANCERS GROW AND SPREAD

The various stages in the development and spread of a cancerous tumor are shown below. The site where cancer originally develops is known as a primary tumor. Until a primary tumor reaches the size of about 1 gram, it cannot be detected. By this time, cells from the original tumor site may have spread to other parts of the body to form secondary tumors. This process is known as metastasis; it occurs because cancer cells have the ability to travel through the lymphatic system and the bloodstream.

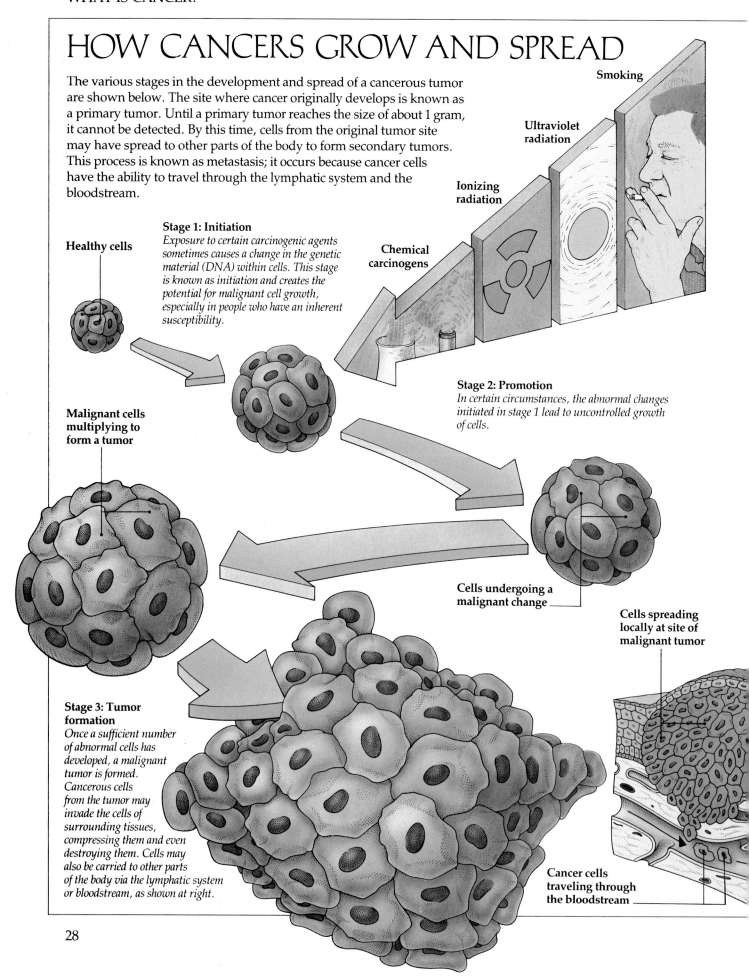

Smoking

Ultraviolet radiation

Ionizing radiation

Chemical carcinogens

Healthy cells

Stage 1: Initiation
Exposure to certain carcinogenic agents sometimes causes a change in the genetic material (DNA) within cells. This stage is known as initiation and creates the potential for malignant cell growth, especially in people who have an inherent susceptibility.

Stage 2: Promotion
In certain circumstances, the abnormal changes initiated in stage 1 lead to uncontrolled growth of cells.

Malignant cells multiplying to form a tumor

Cells undergoing a malignant change

Cells spreading locally at site of malignant tumor

Stage 3: Tumor formation
Once a sufficient number of abnormal cells has developed, a malignant tumor is formed. Cancerous cells from the tumor may invade the cells of surrounding tissues, compressing them and even destroying them. Cells may also be carried to other parts of the body via the lymphatic system or bloodstream, as shown at right.

Cancer cells traveling through the bloodstream

THE ROUTES OF METASTASIS

LYMPHATIC SPREAD

KEY

○ Primary tumor

⇨ Spread of cancer

°o° Secondary growths

BLOOD SPREAD

Lymph glands

Lymphatic vessels

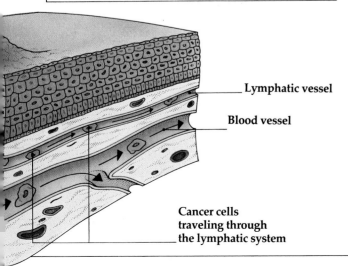

The lymphatic network

Cancerous cells from a primary site may easily enter surrounding lymphatic vessels, which transport them to regional lymph glands and then around the body. Tumor cells may become lodged in lymph glands (eventually forming secondary growths) or may invade tissues supplied by the lymphatic network. Cells may also leave the lymphatic system and enter the bloodstream.

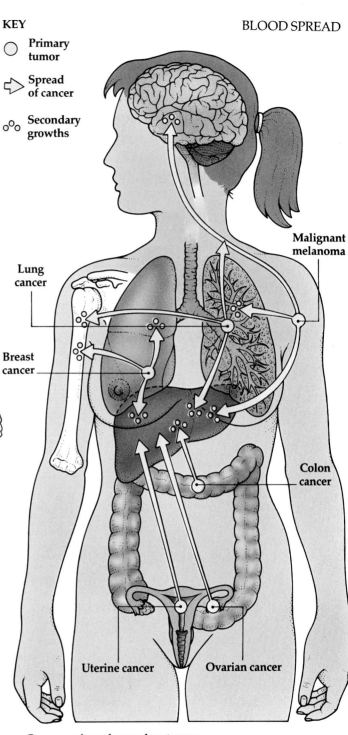

Malignant melanoma

Lung cancer

Breast cancer

Colon cancer

Uterine cancer

Ovarian cancer

Lymphatic vessel

Blood vessel

Cancer cells traveling through the lymphatic system

Common sites of secondary tumors

When an invading cancer encounters a small blood vessel, it can grow through the wall until it reaches the bloodstream. Small collections of cancer cells may then be carried and deposited in other parts of the body to form secondary growths. Certain sites (such as the liver and bones) are more common sites of secondary tumors than others as a result of the arrangement of the blood vessels and the fact that certain tissues seem to provide a better environment than others for growth of cancer cells.

THE EFFECTS OF CANCER

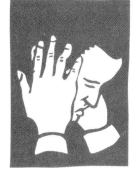

THERE ARE NO SIGNS that can be regarded as typical of cancer. A person may have a large tumor without suffering any obvious symptoms. Even when symptoms do appear, a person may simply feel tired or lacking in energy. That is why many authorities believe that it is important to screen apparently healthy people for cancer. The chance of a cure is improved if the cancer is detected as early as possible.

The effects of malignancy depend on the type and site of the cancer. In some instances, the most obvious effect is the formation of a lump or growth that can be seen or felt. In many cases, there is no visible symptom of the disease but there are physical effects at the site of a tumor. Cancer can also cause widespread, general effects on the body.

Examining a patient for signs of cancer
A physical examination may lead a doctor to consider the possibility of cancer. For example, palpation of the abdomen, shown below, can reveal a possibly malignant tumor that has spread to the liver.

A hidden cause of disease
Sometimes the presence of cancer leads to the development of another recognizable medical condition such as jaundice (shown in the photograph above) or ichthyosis (the dry skin disorder shown at right). It may not always be apparent, however, that cancer is the underlying cause.

GENERAL EFFECTS

Tumor cells release chemical substances, often proteins, that are carried throughout the body by the bloodstream. Some of these substances resemble hormones and can have widespread and severe effects if produced in large quantities. Some tumors manufacture a wide range of these hormonelike substances. Certain cancers of the lung, for instance, can produce hormones that affect the kidneys' ability to control excretion, which can lead to fluid retention. Breast cancers and some lung and kidney tumors can produce hormones that raise the level of blood calcium to a dangerous degree, causing vomiting, dehydration, and coma.

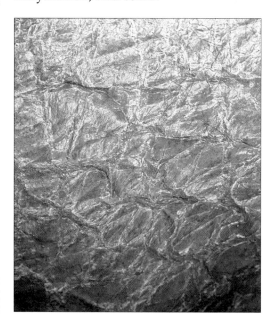

Tumors of the endocrine glands (the pituitary, thyroid, parathyroids, pancreas, adrenals, and sex glands) can, rarely, result in the production of inappropriately and sometimes dangerously large amounts of the hormones normally secreted by these glands. The effect of these hormones is an exaggeration of the normal action of the glands.

Cachexia

In addition to the hormonelike effects, tumors produce a variety of general effects, not all of which are fully understood. These effects include nausea, loss of appetite, anemia, fever, skin rashes, weakness, abnormalities of taste, and severe and progressive weight loss. The end result is often the state known as cachexia, in which so much weight is lost that the patient looks emaciated. Cachexia may result from the tumor using up glucose (the body's energy source) or from malnutrition, bowel obstruction, defective absorption of food, or simply from the loss of appetite that is a common feature of widespread cancer. Cachexia may also occur in people who have small tumors that do not produce any of these effects. The reason why this occurs is not clear.

The cause of death in people with widespread cancer is usually a combination of several factors such as cachexia, infection, internal bleeding, and compromised function of vital tissues by a growing tumor. Of these, infection is probably the most significant cause. Destruction of essential tissues is a less common cause of death.

Visible tumors
In many cases, the first detectable effect of cancer is the development of a lump or growth. In the photograph below, the obvious swelling under the patient's skin is a tumor of the thyroid gland.

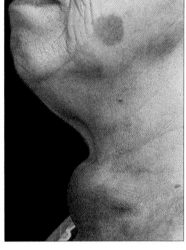

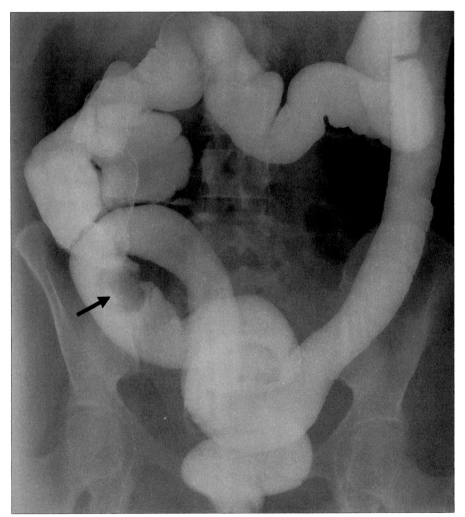

Cancerous polyp in colon
In the color-enhanced X-ray at left, the patient has been given a barium enema to highlight the intestine. A polyp-shaped tumor is visible in the X-ray as a dark area (arrow) in the sigmoid colon. Cancers of the colon may take three forms – flat and ulcerative, polyp-shaped, or encircling. The latter two may eventually obstruct the passage of feces. All three may also lead to abdominal pain, bloating, and blood in the stools. Before obstruction occurs, when the tumor is near the outlet of the bowels, stringlike feces may be produced. This is an important sign of cancer, though it may also occur in the disorder known as irritable colon.

CASE HISTORY
THE DANGERS OF DELAYING DIAGNOSIS

JACQUELINE HAD ALWAYS **been afraid to examine her breasts for changes. For some time she had been under the impression that her breasts no longer looked alike. But she couldn't bring herself to go to her doctor. She was afraid of what he might find. While dressing one day, she noticed that the skin of one breast puckered inward when she raised her arms. After weeks of hesitation, she decided to consult her doctor.**

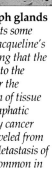

PERSONAL DETAILS
Name Jacqueline Farmer
Age 54
Occupation Fashion designer
Family No history of any major diseases.

MEDICAL BACKGROUND
Jacqueline has been afraid of illness all her life and avoids doctors. She is a nonsmoker and doesn't drink. She is acutely conscious of her appearance and careful of her diet.

THE CONSULTATION
During a physical examination, Jacqueline's doctor discovers an obvious hard lump on the upper and outer side of Jacqueline's right breast. The doctor asks her how long she has had the lump but Jacqueline says she doesn't know be-

cause she hasn't ever examined herself. She says her breasts have always been "lumpy". The doctor is seriously concerned and refers Jacqueline to a surgeon.

THE DIAGNOSIS
The surgeon tells Jacqueline that she probably has BREAST CANCER. He explains that the tumor needs to be biopsied and, if necessary, removed. He explains that the clinical signs indicate that the lump is fixed to the underlying muscle on her chest wall and to the skin above it. That is why the skin is unable to move normally when she raises her arm. Tethering of this kind is a sign of locally spreading cancer.

The surgeon's examination also reveals that Jacqueline has some small, hard, beanlike swellings in the armpit on the same side as the lump. These are lymph glands to which the cancer cells may have spread. A biopsy is performed and then bone and liver scans are done. The scans show no detectable spread of the cancer.

The surgeon tells her that, with treatment, she has a 60 to 75 percent chance of recovery. He explains her disease in more detail and tells Jacqueline that an experienced medical staff with practical experience in helping cancer patients is available to her.

The surgeon tells her that he does not believe in radical surgery but that it is essential to remove all obviously cancerous tissue. Jacqueline will have chemotherapy to help destroy the malignant cells, followed by surgery and radiation. She will also take the antiestrogen drug tamoxifen if estrogen receptors are present in the tumor. This drug is helpful in treating breast cancer in women who have gone

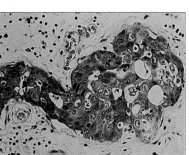

Examining lymph glands
The surgeon detects some swellings under Jacqueline's right arm indicating that the cancer has spread to the lymph glands near the breast. The section of tissue above shows a lymphatic channel blocked by cancer cells that have traveled from a breast tumor. Metastasis of this kind is very common in breast cancer.

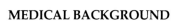

through the menopause because it reduces the chances of cancer spread by neutralizing the female sex hormone estrogen, which encourages the growth of cancer cells.

The surgeon tells Jacqueline that reconstructive surgery on her breast can ultimately restore its appearance. She agrees that nothing could be as bad as wondering about the cancer and gives her consent to the operation.

THE TREATMENT
Jacqueline has a simple mastectomy with removal of all apparently cancerous tissue. Part of the muscle under her breast, invaded by the tumor, also must be removed along with some of the adherent skin. She is given radiation therapy and treated with tamoxifen.

Jacqueline's morale is greatly improved when she is given a breast prosthesis. With her friends' encouragement, she decides to go ahead with reconstructive surgery.

THE OUTCOME
For 2 years Jacqueline remains well, seeing her surgeon regularly for checkups. Then, one day, she trips over a basket of clothes on the floor of her workroom. She is in great pain and is found to have a fracture of her left thighbone. At first, the fracture is thought to be due to osteoporosis but an X-ray reveals the unmistakable signs of secondary bone cancer. A scan shows multiple secondary deposits of cancer in her bones, liver, and other parts of the body. Evidently, cancer cells from her original tumor had spread (metastasized).

The doctors recommend chemotherapy; Jacqueline agrees without hesitation. She is still undergoing treatment and surveillance.

SOME LOCAL EFFECTS OF CANCER

There are many different local effects of cancer. Tumors may become very large and compress or displace surrounding structures. Tumors can erode and damage organs and blood vessels, block tubes, destroy vital functional tissue, form abnormal connections between organs and body cavities, and promote internal bleeding and the production of abnormal quantities of fluid. Below are examples of the possible local effects of some specific cancers.

◆ Cancer of the esophagus may cause such an obstruction that only small quantities of food can enter the stomach. The result may be severe malnutrition. In some cases, liquid but not solid food may pass. The obstruction may result from the tumor protruding into the esophagus or from a ringlike narrowing.

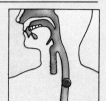

◆ The front wall of part of the rectum is in close contact with the back wall of the vagina. A rectal tumor in this location may break through the vaginal wall so that feces and intestinal gas can pass into the vagina. Such a cancerous tumor can also break through into the bladder, causing urinary infection, secondary damage to the kidneys, and gas in the urine.

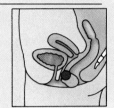

◆ It is common for lung cancer to grow to obstruct one of the small bronchial tubes leading to a lobule or lobe of the lung. Such obstruction may lead to reduced lung efficiency and invariably causes collapse of the segment of the lung beyond the obstruction. Rarely, lung cancer can erode a large artery, leading to severe and possibly uncontrollable bleeding into the lung accompanied by the coughing up of bloodstained sputum or pure blood.

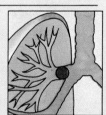

◆ Cancer of the prostate occasionally obstructs the outflow of urine so that only a small amount of urine is able to be passed at a time and only when the bladder is very full and at maximum tension. This causes repeated attempts to urinate at short intervals and great disturbance of sleep. Such outflow obstruction leads to severe pressure in the bladder and ureters and can eventually result in loss of kidney function.

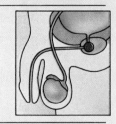

◆ Cancers may encroach on nerves and destroy their function, so that the muscles supplied by the nerves are paralyzed. This commonly involves damage to one of the nerves that control the vocal cords. These nerves loop down into the chest and are often involved in cancer of the lung. The nerve damage may lead to a severe hoarseness due to paralysis of one of the vocal cords.

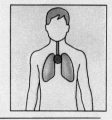

◆ Cancer of the head of the pancreas commonly causes obstruction of the pancreatic and bile ducts at the point at which these ducts open together into the small intestine. This has several effects. The digestive juices from the pancreas cannot get into the intestine so digestion and absorption are affected and the enzymes trapped in the pancreas may start to digest the organ itself. Blockage of the bile duct causes bile pigments to accumulate in the liver and then in the blood, leading to progressively worsening jaundice from staining of the skin by bile.

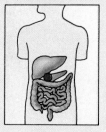

CHAPTER THREE

CAUSES AND PREVENTION

ALTHOUGH IT IS ONLY rarely possible to be certain of the cause of a particular cancer, we do know a lot about the factors that influence the development of cancer in general. In the early days of X-ray technology, workers had no idea that X-rays were in any way dangerous, and they made no attempt to protect themselves from the radiation. Cancer, especially of the hands, developed in almost all of these pioneers, and many of them died of it. In a similar way, workers employed to paint the dials of clocks and watches with luminous paint containing radium used to "point" their fine paintbrushes by putting them into their mouths. Scores of these workers later died of cancers of the tongue, jaw, and bones.

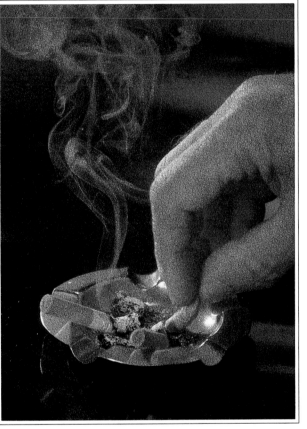

Many substances were discovered to induce skin cancer, including soot, tar, creosote, pitch, and a variety of mineral oils. When cheap shale oil was widely used to lubricate the high-speed spindles of the early cotton mills, the garments of the mill workers were kept soaking wet by a fine spray of oil. As a consequence, skin cancers developed in many of them. The wrinkled skin of the scrotum was particularly susceptible to cancer because the oil tended to remain there for longer periods.

Today, thousands more substances are known to be capable of inducing cancer. These include chemicals in tobacco and tobacco smoke; alcohol (especially if used in conjunction with tobacco); materials or chemicals used in industry, such as asbestos and vinyl chloride; and certain drugs, such as synthetic estrogens. A small number of viruses, as well as certain substances in some foods, are also known or suspected to be carcinogens. And frequent exposure to strong sunlight is a significant cause of skin cancer. All these carcinogenic agents are thought to act by initiating changes in body cells, specifically in the genetic programs that control cell growth and multiplication.

In this chapter we look at a range of life-style factors and the common agents in our environment that are known to cause or have been associated with cancer – aspects of the diet, tobacco, chemical carcinogens, radiation, sunlight, viruses, medications, and sexual behavior. The final section gives a realistic overview of what each of us can do to reduce his or her cancer risk. As noted in this section, quitting smoking – or even better, never starting to smoke – is by far the most important anticancer step that anyone can take.

CANCER AND THE DOUBLE HELIX

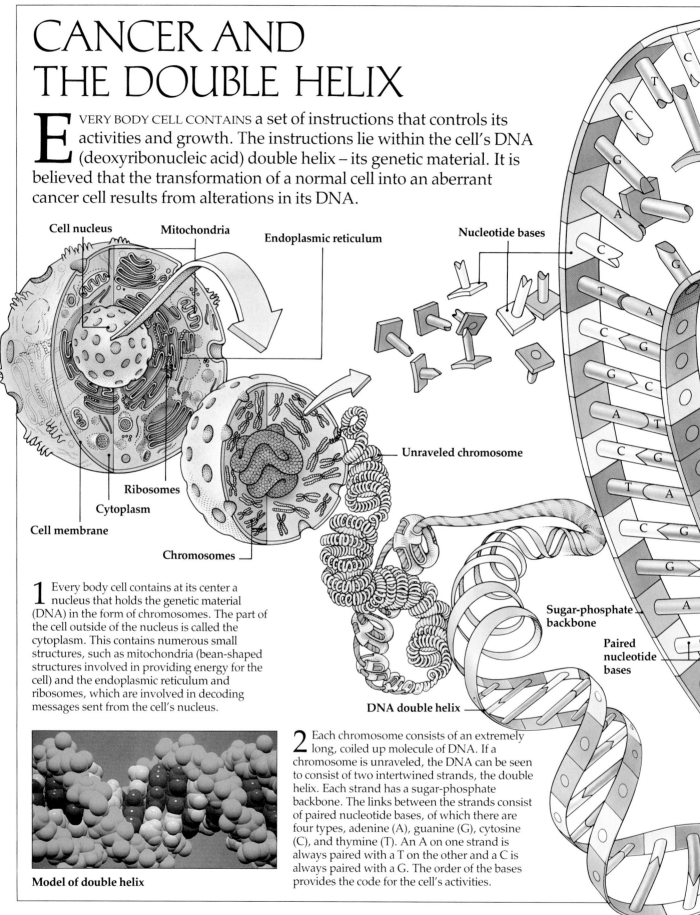

E VERY BODY CELL CONTAINS a set of instructions that controls its activities and growth. The instructions lie within the cell's DNA (deoxyribonucleic acid) double helix – its genetic material. It is believed that the transformation of a normal cell into an aberrant cancer cell results from alterations in its DNA.

Cell nucleus

Mitochondria

Endoplasmic reticulum

Nucleotide bases

Unraveled chromosome

Ribosomes

Cytoplasm

Cell membrane

Chromosomes

Sugar-phosphate backbone

Paired nucleotide bases

DNA double helix

1 Every body cell contains at its center a nucleus that holds the genetic material (DNA) in the form of chromosomes. The part of the cell outside of the nucleus is called the cytoplasm. This contains numerous small structures, such as mitochondria (bean-shaped structures involved in providing energy for the cell) and the endoplasmic reticulum and ribosomes, which are involved in decoding messages sent from the cell's nucleus.

Model of double helix

2 Each chromosome consists of an extremely long, coiled up molecule of DNA. If a chromosome is unraveled, the DNA can be seen to consist of two intertwined strands, the double helix. Each strand has a sugar-phosphate backbone. The links between the strands consist of paired nucleotide bases, of which there are four types, adenine (A), guanine (G), cytosine (C), and thymine (T). An A on one strand is always paired with a T on the other and a C is always paired with a G. The order of the bases provides the code for the cell's activities.

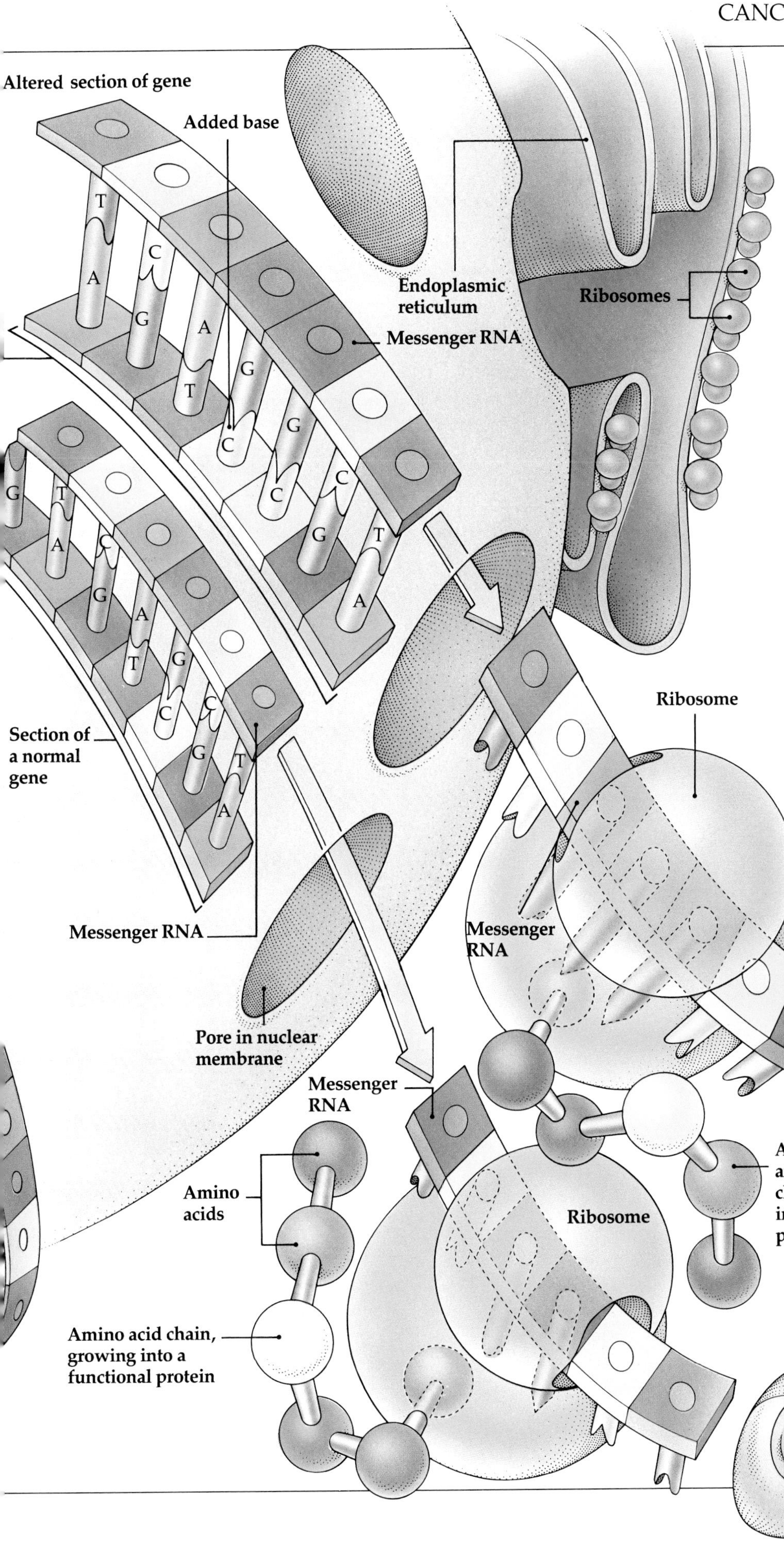

Altered section of gene

Added base

T
A
C
G
A
G
G
G
C
C
G
T
A

Endoplasmic reticulum

Ribosomes

Messenger RNA

G
T
A
C
G
A
T
G
C
G
C
G
T
A

Section of a normal gene

Messenger RNA

Pore in nuclear membrane

Ribosome

Messenger RNA

Messenger RNA

Amino acids

Amino acid chain, growing into a functional protein

Ribosome

Altered amino acid chain, forming into an altered protein

3 For a section of DNA (a gene) to be decoded by the cell, the relevant section of double helix must unravel. One strand acts as a template for a messenger molecule – messenger RNA (ribonucleic acid) – to be formed. The messenger RNA passes out of the nucleus and is latched onto by a decoding particle, called a ribosome. This helps translate the order of the bases on the messenger RNA molecule into a string of amino acids, which build up to form a protein molecule. Proteins then act to determine a cell's activities.

4 Here, two strands of messenger RNA are being formed, passing out of the nucleus, and being decoded. One has been formed from a section of a normal gene, the other from a gene that has been slightly altered (with the addition of a single extra nucleotide base) through the effect of a carcinogenic agent. Decoding of the first strand of RNA leads to the formation of a normal, functional protein; decoding of the other RNA strand leads to the formation of an altered protein. This alteration may lead to a change in the functioning and activities of the cell.

5 Cells that have undergone alterations to their genetic material may begin to function and divide in an aberrant way – possibly leading to cancer.

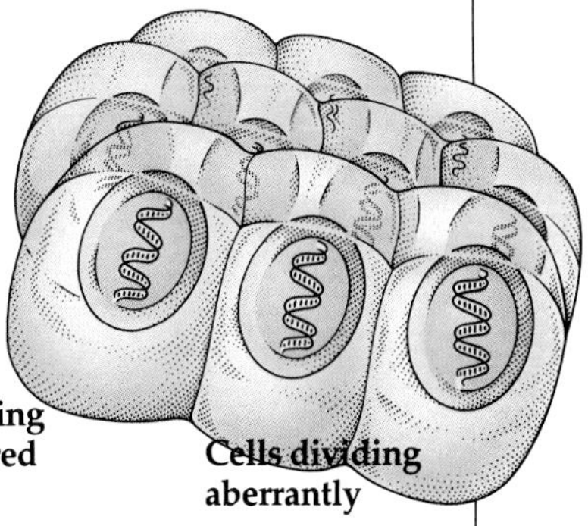

Cells dividing aberrantly

6 Cells that have suffered no alteration, or minimal alteration, to their DNA continue to divide and function normally.

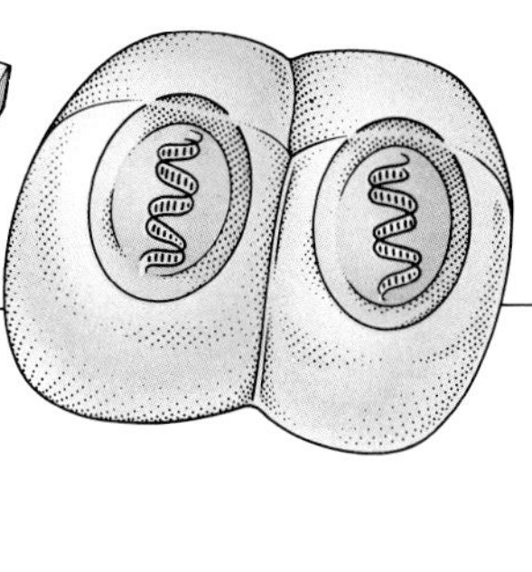

Cells dividing normally

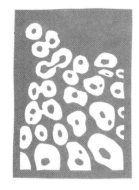

WHAT CAUSES CANCER?

THE THEORY OF ONCOGENES is widely accepted as an explanation for the underlying mechanism of the cause of cancer. It states that alterations inside the genes that control cell growth and division, given a triggering factor, lead to a loss of control over growth and thus to cancer. Genes affected in this way are called oncogenes.

As explained in CANCER AND THE DOUBLE HELIX (pages 36 and 37), it is now accepted that cancer results from alterations in the genetic material within cells. However, not all genetic alterations are cancer-causing. Scientists today strongly suspect that only a minority of alterations – those that activate certain genes called oncogenes – are important.

THE GENETIC LINK

Every cell in the body contains the same genes, of which there are some 50,000 to 100,000 in all. Cells use only those genes relevant to their specific function, and the rest are suppressed. Oncogenes can be thought of as genes that are normally

THE THEORY OF ONCOGENES

Within the DNA (genetic material) of each cell, it is theorized that there are certain genes concerned solely with promotion of cell growth and multiplication. For much of the time, these proto-oncogenes are switched off (are inactive). If the proto-oncogenes become permanently switched on (become active) as a result of

changes in the genetic material brought about by the action of cancer-causing agents, a normal cell may become transformed into a cell that grows and divides abnormally. Other genes, called antioncogenes, suppress abnormal growth. When they are turned off, cells may grow abnormally.

Normal growth
Healthy cells divide in an orderly, regulated, and restrained way – growing and multiplying only enough to replace cells lost as a result of aging or injury.

Mildly abnormal growth (dysplasia)
If one or two oncogenes in a cell are affected by cancer-causing agents acting on the genetic material, the cell and its descendants may begin to grow and divide in a mildly aberrant way.

Malignant growth
Further action of carcinogens on cells that are already mildly abnormal may activate more oncogenes, until a stage is reached where one or more cells begin to multiply in a highly aberrant and chaotic way, leading to the formation of a malignant tumor.

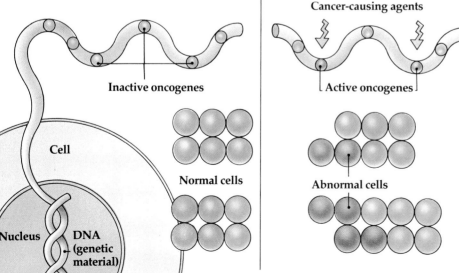

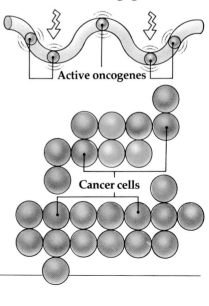

Inactive oncogenes

Cell

Normal cells

Nucleus

DNA (genetic material)

Cancer-causing agents

Active oncogenes

Abnormal cells

Cancer-causing agents

Active oncogenes

Cancer cells

HOW GROWTH FACTORS CAN CAUSE CANCER

The normal cell
Growth factors trigger receptors on cell surfaces, which send messages into the cell, stimulating it to divide.

In a cancer cell
Growth factors may be inappropriately secreted from the cell. These factors stimulate the receptors and provoke division.

Alternatively, a receptor may be damaged and send out secondary messages telling the cell to divide all the time.

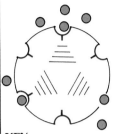 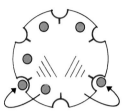 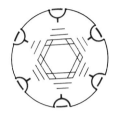

KEY

Receptor ⅄ Message into cell ☰ Growth factor ● Damaged receptor ⅄

THE TIME SCALE

The transformation process that changes a healthy cell into a cancerous one seems to take a long time. In many such cases, the body's natural defense system identifies the cell as cancerous and destroys it. Even when a cell is transformed into a cancer cell and manages to dodge the immune system, it must divide many, many times before its descendants are numerous enough to form a tumor big enough to be detected. Scientists estimate that a typical breast cancer tumor, for example, may have to grow for more than a decade before it becomes detectable.

suppressed except during phases of rapid growth. If sufficient numbers become inappropriately or permanently "switched on," however, they may transform a normal cell into an aberrant cancer cell (see THE THEORY OF ONCOGENES at left).

TRIGGER FACTORS

More than 20 oncogenes have been identified. The outside factors that switch them into action are also being identified. Some of these are known, such as the tarlike substances in tobacco smoke, nuclear radiation, X-rays, the ultraviolet rays in sunlight, and a growing list of natural and industrial chemicals.

It seems probable that more than one oncogene must be switched on before a cell or group of cells becomes sufficiently abnormal to produce a malignant tumor. Furthermore, the carcinogenic process appears to consist of many steps and is divisible into at least two stages – initiation, which appears to be a rapid and irreversible event, and promotion, which takes longer and is at least partially reversible. Different carcinogenic agents may be involved in the two stages.

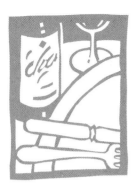

FOOD, ALCOHOL, AND CANCER

IETARY HABITS ARE estimated to be responsible for up to 35 percent of cancer-related deaths in the US, and alcohol use for another 3 percent. Although many of the links between food, alcohol, and cancer are not fully understood or proven, it is recognized that individual control of food and alcohol intake offers an important opportunity to reduce the incidence of several types of cancer.

Research studies of the relationship between diet and cancer worldwide suggest that the incidence of some cancers could be reduced in the US by introducing changes in the types of foods that are eaten, the ways in which the foods are prepared, and the quantities in which foods are consumed. Furthermore, the studies suggest that moderation in the consumption of alcohol is an essential requirement in the prevention of specific cancers. Moderation is particularly important when alcohol intake is accompanied by smoking.

CARCINOGENS IN FOOD

At present, very few recognized carcinogens (cancer-producing substances) are likely to enter the American food supply. However, one possibility is the powerful carcinogen aflatoxin, a poison produced by the mold *Aspergillus flavus*, which grows on damp peanuts and other crops. Effective quality control and preserving techniques have reduced aflatoxin contamination to very low levels in the US and most other developed countries.

Benzopyrene in foods
Benzopyrene, a substance found on the charred surfaces of charcoal-broiled foods and throughout smoke-cured products, has been shown to cause cancer in animals but its effect on humans is unknown. The American Cancer Society recommends that foods that are charcoal-broiled or smoke-cured be eaten only in moderation. If you wish to charcoal-broil, use lean cuts of meat and wrap the meat or fish in foil to reduce contact with smoke and flame. Foods should be fried or grilled at temperatures below 300°F (150°C).

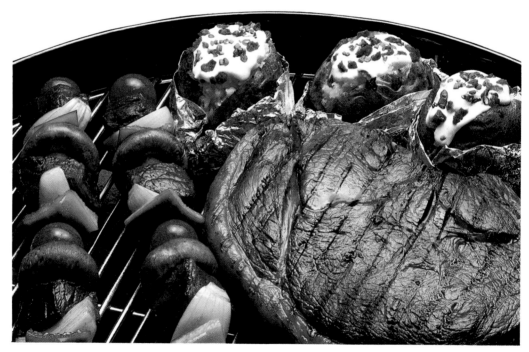

Some chemicals in food are suspected of being converted by the body into carcinogens. Among these are the nitrates and nitrites used to preserve meat and sausage, which may be converted in the stomach to carcinogenic nitrosamines. Ascorbic acid (vitamin C) is now often added to such foods to reduce the risk. Nitrosamines may also be produced by smoking or overcooking animal protein.

Salt and spices

Preserving fish by drying and salting is also considered potentially harmful; the high incidence of cancer of the back of the nose (nasopharyngeal cancer) in the Far East may be associated with salted fish in the diet. Links are suspected between stomach cancer and highly spiced food, highly acidic foods such as pickles, and the concentrated alcohol in hard liquor, but these links are not proved. Except for a few instances, causative agents have not been identified in cured, pickled, or smoked foods.

OBESITY

To determine whether obesity affects the incidence of cancer, the American Cancer Society monitored 1 million people and recorded the incidence of cancers of the cervix, breast, and kidney in women and cancer of the colon in men. The society concluded that people 40 percent or more above the ideal weight for their height are twice as likely to die of these cancers as people of normal weight.

However, these findings do not prove that cancers are directly caused by obesity. There are socioeconomic and environmental factors associated with obesity that may be instrumental in the higher incidence of cancer. Also, obesity may delay the diagnosis of cancer, increasing the death rate for that reason alone. Furthermore, people substantially below average weight also have a raised mortality from cancer, indicating that the relationship to weight is complex.

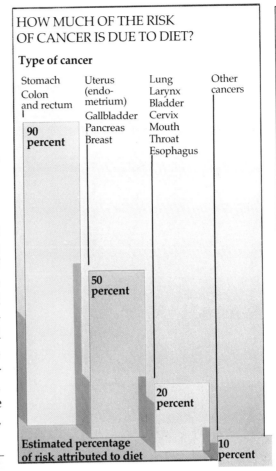

HOW MUCH OF THE RISK OF CANCER IS DUE TO DIET?

Type of cancer

Stomach Colon and rectum — Uterus (endometrium) Gallbladder Pancreas Breast — Lung Larynx Bladder Cervix Mouth Throat Esophagus — Other cancers

90 percent

50 percent

20 percent

10 percent

Estimated percentage of risk attributed to diet

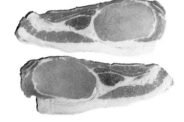

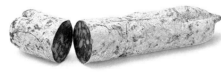

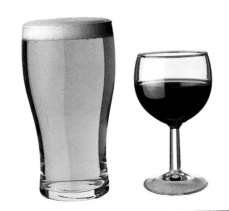

DIETARY RECOMMENDATIONS

In 1988, the Surgeon General's Report on Nutrition and Health noted that a variety of agencies have issued dietary recommendations as part of a nationwide campaign to reduce the incidence of all cancers. The National Cancer Institute's dietary guidelines are:
◆ Reduce fat intake to 30 percent or less of calories.
◆ Increase fiber intake to 20 to 30 grams daily.
◆ Include a variety of vegetables and fruits in your daily diet.
◆ Avoid obesity.
◆ Consume alcoholic beverages in moderation, if at all.
◆ Minimize consumption of salt-cured, pickled, and smoked foods.

Dietary moderation
Eating a wide variety of fresh foods of all types is the best safeguard against diet-related disease, including cancer. A moderate consumption of smoked or salt-cured foods (such as bacon) and nitrate-preserved foods (such as sausage), and a moderate intake of alcohol (one or two glasses a day at the most, with at least several alcohol-free days a week) are unlikely to cause cancer in healthy people who do not smoke.

ASK YOUR DOCTOR
FOOD, ALCOHOL, AND CANCER

Q **Can a vitamin-rich diet, or the use of vitamins, help reduce the risk of cancer?**

A There is some evidence that people who eat diets rich in vitamins A and C have lower rates of cancer. In theory, vitamins A, C, and E could prevent, or help reverse, damage to body cells caused by carcinogens. However, studies have been inconclusive.

Q **My father has been a heavy drinker for many years. Is he at increased risk of liver cancer?**

A A prolonged high intake of alcohol causes liver cirrhosis, and some people with cirrhosis go on to get liver cancer. But alcohol, especially when coupled with cigarette smoking, is also linked to other cancers that are much more common than liver cancer.

Q **Could cancer be caused by eating too much fat? If so, by what mechanism?**

A High-fat diets increase the bile acids and cholesterol in the feces. Some evidence suggests that cholesterol and bile acids are changed by bacteria in the intestine into other chemicals, some of which could be carcinogenic.

Q **What are cruciferous vegetables and how might they guard against cancer?**

A Cruciferous vegetables include cabbage, brussels sprouts, broccoli, kohlrabi, and cauliflower. They have been associated with a reduction in the risk of cancers of the gastrointestinal and respiratory tracts.

HOW DOES FIBER PREVENT COLON CANCER?

People who eat high-fiber diets have a much lower incidence of cancer of the colon and rectum than those who eat low-fiber diets. Exactly why this is so is unknown, but it is thought to occur because a regular intake of fiber speeds the passage of fecal matter through the digestive tract.

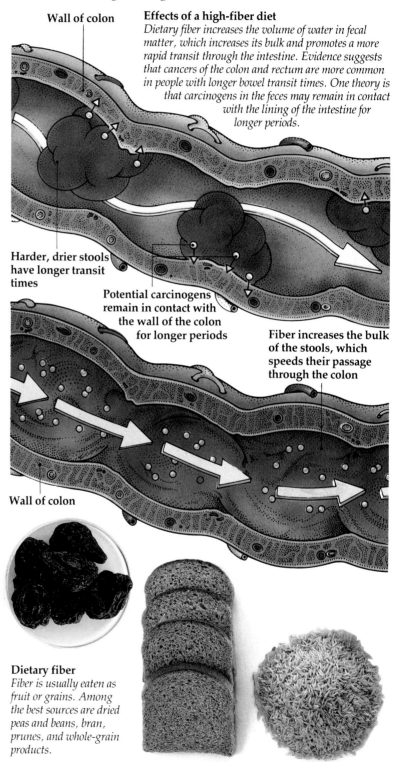

Wall of colon

Effects of a high-fiber diet
Dietary fiber increases the volume of water in fecal matter, which increases its bulk and promotes a more rapid transit through the intestine. Evidence suggests that cancers of the colon and rectum are more common in people with longer bowel transit times. One theory is that carcinogens in the feces may remain in contact with the lining of the intestine for longer periods.

Harder, drier stools have longer transit times

Potential carcinogens remain in contact with the wall of the colon for longer periods

Fiber increases the bulk of the stools, which speeds their passage through the colon

Wall of colon

Dietary fiber
Fiber is usually eaten as fruit or grains. Among the best sources are dried peas and beans, bran, prunes, and whole-grain products.

DIETARY FATS AND DIETARY FIBER

While a 1988 report on nutrition and health noted inconsistencies in data relating dietary fat to cancer causation, studies to date suggest that dietary fat plays a role in some types of cancer. One example can be seen in the descendants of people who emigrate from areas of low fat intake, such as Japan, to areas of higher fat intake, such as the US. These individuals have a higher incidence of certain cancers than exists in their country of origin. The picture is complicated, however, by the fact that diets high in fat are generally low in fiber; there remains a possibility that diets low in fiber, just as much as diets high in fat, may cause the cancers.

Cancer of the large intestine (the colon) is a common cause of death in developed countries, such as the US, yet it is rare in less-developed communities. However, evidence of a direct link between colon cancer and fat and fiber consumption has been inconclusive. It is also difficult to measure the amounts of each of the types of fiber in foods, so the effects of the different fiber types on the incidence of bowel cancer are largely unknown.

ALCOHOL ABUSE

A high intake of alcoholic beverages increases the risk of cancers of the mouth, throat, larynx, and esophagus. Drinks that contain alcohol in a more concentrated form (such as hard liquor) are more likely to have an adverse effect. But it is not known whether the responsible agent is alcohol itself or any of the more than 400 other chemicals contained in alcoholic beverages. Highly significant is the synergistic effect of alcohol and tobacco. The risk factor created by using alcohol and tobacco together is greater than the sum of the risk factors of each used on its own.

COFFEE AND CANCER OF THE PANCREAS

The interpretation of population studies requires great caution. Some years ago, researchers noted that patients with pancreatic cancer drank a lot of coffee. This led the researchers to implicate coffee – though cautiously – as a causative factor. Further evidence, however, suggested that the coffee drinking was due to thirst caused by the pancreatic disease.

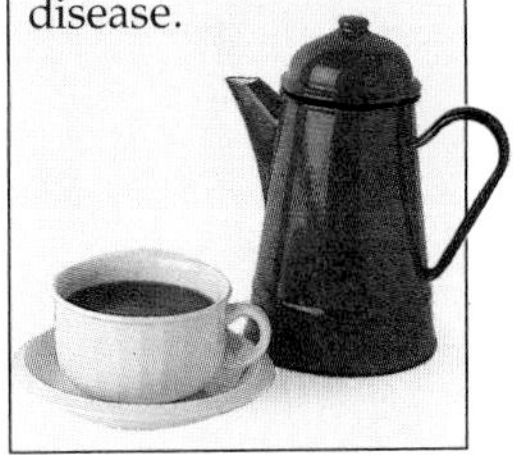

ALCOHOL, SMOKING, AND CANCER

The chart below shows the results of a study that assessed the risk of esophageal cancer for four ranges of alcohol intake, to which were added four ranges of cigarette use. The study showed that people who drink and smoke heavily are at enormously increased risk of esophageal cancer.

Daily cigarette intake	
Under 15	Under 40
Under 25	40 or more

Daily alcohol intake (g = grams)	
0 to 40 g	81 to 120 g
41 to 80 g	121 g or more

Risk of cancer of the esophagus relative to risk of a person who drinks less than 40 grams of alcohol and smokes fewer than 15 cigarettes a day

×149.3
×130.7
×87.1
×64.0
×49.8
×35.5
×11.7 ×13.6 ×12.4
×7.8
×7.3 ×8.4 ×8.8
×1.0 ×3.4 ×3.8

Up to four 4-ounce glasses of wine or three 1½-ounce shots of hard liquor

Up to one bottle and two 4-ounce glasses of wine or six 1½-ounce shots of hard liquor

Up to two bottles of wine or nine 1½-ounce shots of hard liquor

More than two bottles of wine or nine 1½-ounce shots of hard liquor

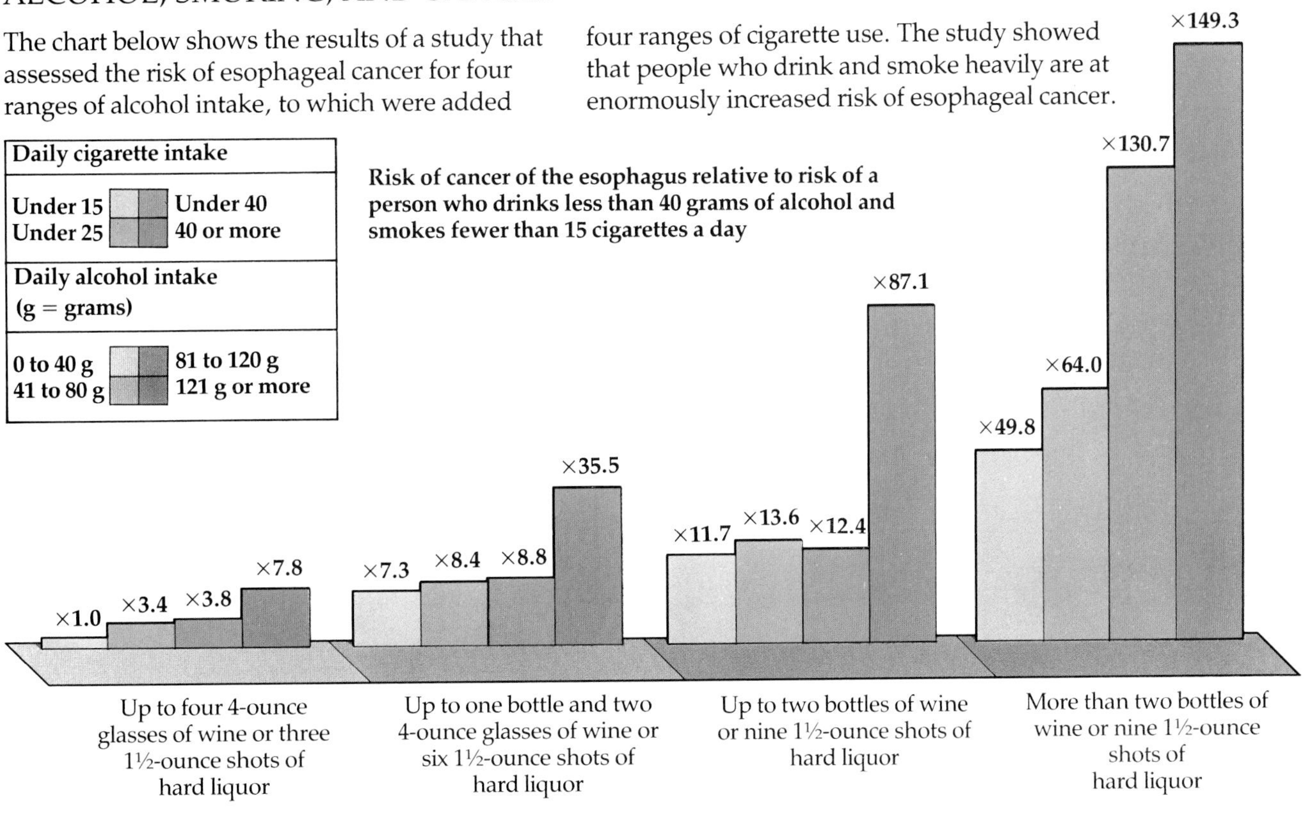

SMOKING AND CANCER

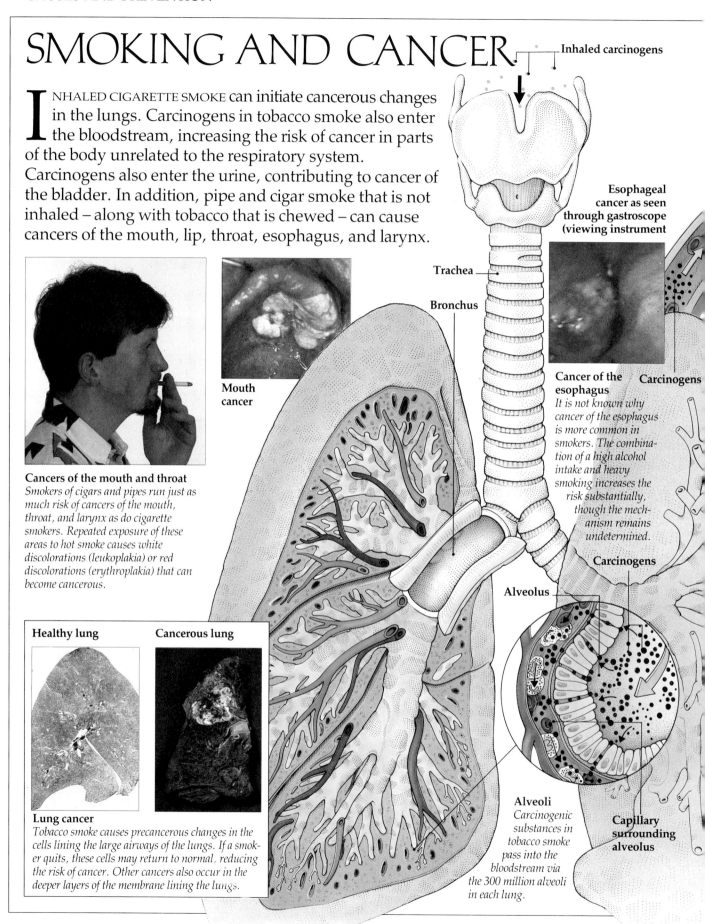

Inhaled carcinogens

INHALED CIGARETTE SMOKE can initiate cancerous changes in the lungs. Carcinogens in tobacco smoke also enter the bloodstream, increasing the risk of cancer in parts of the body unrelated to the respiratory system. Carcinogens also enter the urine, contributing to cancer of the bladder. In addition, pipe and cigar smoke that is not inhaled – along with tobacco that is chewed – can cause cancers of the mouth, lip, throat, esophagus, and larynx.

Esophageal cancer as seen through gastroscope (viewing instrument

Mouth cancer

Trachea

Bronchus

Cancer of the esophagus
It is not known why cancer of the esophagus is more common in smokers. The combination of a high alcohol intake and heavy smoking increases the risk substantially, though the mechanism remains undetermined.

Carcinogens

Cancers of the mouth and throat
Smokers of cigars and pipes run just as much risk of cancers of the mouth, throat, and larynx as do cigarette smokers. Repeated exposure of these areas to hot smoke causes white discolorations (leukoplakia) or red discolorations (erythroplakia) that can become cancerous.

Carcinogens

Alveolus

Healthy lung

Cancerous lung

Lung cancer
Tobacco smoke causes precancerous changes in the cells lining the large airways of the lungs. If a smoker quits, these cells may return to normal, reducing the risk of cancer. Other cancers also occur in the deeper layers of the membrane lining the lungs.

Alveoli
Carcinogenic substances in tobacco smoke pass into the bloodstream via the 300 million alveoli in each lung.

Capillary surrounding alveolus

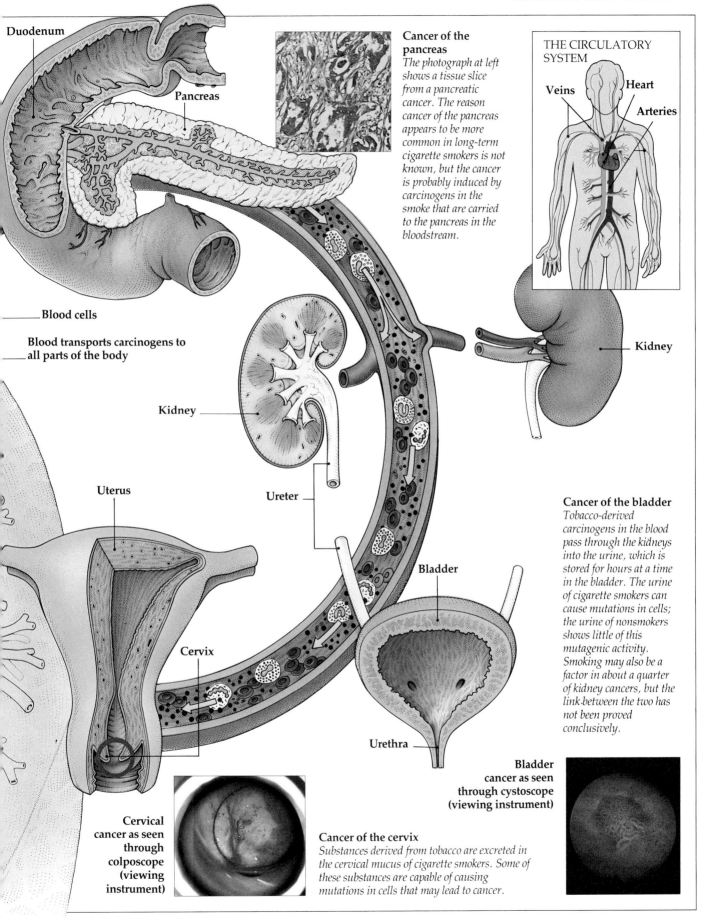

Duodenum

Pancreas

Cancer of the pancreas
The photograph at left shows a tissue slice from a pancreatic cancer. The reason cancer of the pancreas appears to be more common in long-term cigarette smokers is not known, but the cancer is probably induced by carcinogens in the smoke that are carried to the pancreas in the bloodstream.

THE CIRCULATORY SYSTEM

Veins

Heart

Arteries

Blood cells

Blood transports carcinogens to all parts of the body

Kidney

Kidney

Uterus

Ureter

Cervix

Bladder

Urethra

Cancer of the bladder
Tobacco-derived carcinogens in the blood pass through the kidneys into the urine, which is stored for hours at a time in the bladder. The urine of cigarette smokers can cause mutations in cells; the urine of nonsmokers shows little of this mutagenic activity. Smoking may also be a factor in about a quarter of kidney cancers, but the link between the two has not been proved conclusively.

Cervical cancer as seen through colposcope (viewing instrument)

Bladder cancer as seen through cystoscope (viewing instrument)

Cancer of the cervix
Substances derived from tobacco are excreted in the cervical mucus of cigarette smokers. Some of these substances are capable of causing mutations in cells that may lead to cancer.

45

PASSIVE SMOKING

Breathing in smoke from other people's cigarettes is known as passive smoking. Nonsmokers who are regularly exposed to tobacco smoke have a risk of cancer 10 to 30 percent higher than that of nonsmokers. In young children, the harmful effects of passive smoking are even greater.

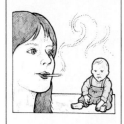

The smoking habit takes a heavy toll – 350,000 people in the US die of smoking-related diseases each year and, of these, about 135,000 die of cancer. Smoking causes a large percentage of cancers in several organs. For example, if all the smokers in America quit tomorrow, the incidence of lung cancer in the US would eventually drop by 85 percent.

Tobacco smoke, particularly cigarette smoke, is a complex mixture of more than 3,000 distinguishable substances. Several of these substances are converted by the body into cancer-causing (carcinogenic) agents. As a result, smoking can initiate cancers in many different organs in the body.

Probably the most important of these substances is called benzopyrene. During metabolism in the body this substance is changed chemically into more than 40 other substances. One of these is diol epoxide, a highly carcinogenic substance that is capable of causing mutations in DNA; diol epoxide is found chemically bound to DNA in the cells of cigarette smokers.

The rate at which smokers metabolize substances such as benzopyrene is determined genetically – some people have more enzymes that carry out this function than others. Cancers are seen most often in people who metabolize these substances at a rapid rate.

TOBACCO-RELATED CANCERS

The risk of getting cancer from cigarette smoking varies according to the number of cigarettes smoked per day, the age at which smoking began, the amount of tar in the cigarettes, the depth of inhalation, and several other factors.

HOW DOES SMOKING CAUSE LUNG CANCER?

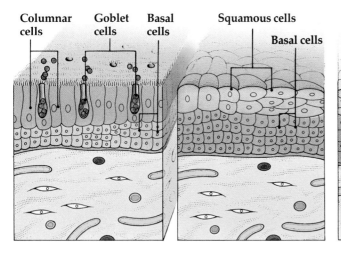

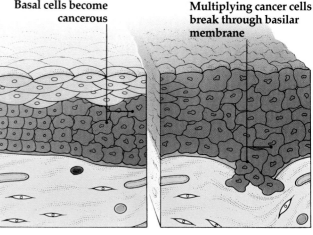

Columnar cells **Goblet cells** **Basal cells** **Squamous cells** **Basal cells** **Basal cells become cancerous** **Multiplying cancer cells break through basilar membrane**

1 Most so-called lung cancers actually occur in the bronchi, the tubes through which air passes into the lungs. The bronchi are lined by tall cells, known as columnar cells, that are covered by fine hairs, or cilia. The bronchi are lubricated by mucus that is produced by goblet cells.

2 Over a period of time, smoking causes these cells, especially those at the angle of the bronchial branches, to undergo a change known as dysplasia. The columnar cells lose their cilia and become more cube-shaped, progressing to a flattened, squamous type of cell similar to those on the surface of the skin.

3 During this time, replacement cells and cilia are being generated by the basal layer to replace those mutated or destroyed by the tobacco smoke. However, in certain circumstances, regeneration fails to prevent the spread of squamous cells. The underlying basal cells multiply at an increased rate and some transform into cancer cells.

4 The cancer cells multiply quickly, replacing the healthy basal cells and the overlying squamous cells. Eventually, the growing cancer breaks through the membrane underlying the cells and spreads into the connective tissue lying beneath. The tissues of adjacent organs soon are affected.

Mouth and throat

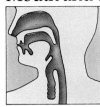

Cancer of the mouth (including the lip, gum, and tongue) and cancer of the throat tend to be related to oral contact with tobacco (mainly smoking or tobacco chewing) and to alcohol consumption. They are very rare in people who don't smoke, use tobacco, or drink. In the case of tobacco chewers, the cancer tends to develop where the tobacco wad is habitually held in the mouth. The Oriental practice of smoking with the burning end of the cigarette inside the mouth causes cancer of the palate, an otherwise very rare condition.

Lung

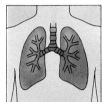

Cigarette smoking is the main cause of lung cancer, and lung cancer develops in about 10 percent of smokers. Whether or not a smoker will get lung cancer is governed by many factors, principally the age at which smoking began and the number of cigarettes smoked per day. The amount of tar and nicotine in cigarettes may also be factors. Alcohol and agents such as asbestos interact synergistically with tobacco smoke to produce an even higher risk.

Esophagus

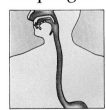

Cancer of the esophagus kills more than 8,500 Americans every year. People who smoke two packages of cigarettes a day may have up to 12 times the risk of esophageal cancer as nonsmokers. One reason for this may be that carcinogens from tobacco are carried into the esophagus by saliva. Heavy alcohol consumption combined with heavy smoking increases the risk dramatically (see ALCOHOL, SMOKING, AND CANCER on page 43).

Pancreas

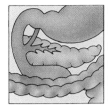

Cancer of the pancreas is two to three times as common in people who smoke heavily as it is in nonsmokers. It is not known why the pancreas, in particular, is vulnerable to smoking-related cancers, although it is believed that dietary factors (including a heavy intake of alcohol and a high intake of fat) may play some part.

Cervix

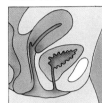

The most significant cause of cancer of the cervix is almost certainly one or two strains of human papillomavirus (the cause of genital warts). The incidence of this cancer increases in proportion to the number of sexual partners. In addition, cigarette smokers have a higher incidence of cervical cancer than nonsmokers.

Bladder

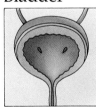

Cigarette smoke contains a minute quantity of the most powerful carcinogen known, naphthylamine. In 1949 a British factory distilling this industrial antioxidant ceased production after cancer of the bladder developed in all of the 19 men who worked there. The carcinogen also caused bladder cancers in men involved in the manufacture of coal gas. It is not known whether the relatively high incidence of bladder cancer in smokers is due to naphthylamine or to other factors. Superficial bladder cancers may respond positively to destruction with a high-frequency current. Chemotherapy or immunotherapy are also used. Bladder cancer has a tendency to recur and surgical removal of the entire bladder is sometimes required when the tumor has spread through the bladder wall.

CAN THE CANCER RISK OF SMOKING BE CALCULATED?

The link between smoking and an increased risk of cancer is firmly established for some sites in the body, including the lungs, mouth, throat, larynx, esophagus, and bladder. A higher risk is also suspected in relation to cancers of the pancreas, kidney, and stomach, but the evidence for these is less conclusive. As an example (see the figures below), the risk of lung cancer in smokers is 10 times the risk of cancer in nonsmokers.

Cancer site	Risk factor
Lungs	10
Larynx	8
Mouth	4
Throat	4
Esophagus	3
Bladder	2
Pancreas	2
Kidney	1.5
Stomach	1.5

CHEMICAL CAUSES OF CANCER

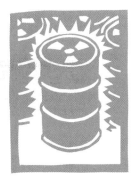

RESEARCH HAS REVEALED that exposure to certain chemicals increases the risk of cancers. Chemicals are, in fact, the largest group of established carcinogens. Although many chemical carcinogens have been positively identified, it is possible that there are others whose dangers have yet to be confirmed.

Pollution and cancer
Studies suggest that, when the atmosphere is heavily polluted by coal smoke, the chemicals it contains may contribute to higher levels of lung cancer. Attempts have been made to reduce air pollution in urban areas, thereby lowering the risk of disease. However, people who live near the source of industrial carcinogens may be at increased risk.

Awareness of the potential hazards of chemical exposure has led to vigorous attempts to reduce the risks of cancer from this source. However, modern technology and the widespread use of chemicals will inevitably bring new chemical carcinogens.

CHEMICALS IN THE ENVIRONMENT

Many people are exposed to chemicals in the home, at work, or in the environment. Potentially dangerous chemicals are sometimes released into the air, dumped in lakes, oceans, or rivers, or buried underground. Residues may eventually infiltrate our air, water, and food supplies.

The idea that pollution might cause cancer has been of increasing concern ever since it was discovered that the incidence of lung cancer tended to be higher in cities than in the country and that the combustion products of fossil fuels, such as coal, contain carcinogens. Assessing the risks using population studies is a retrospective process; people must be exposed to cancer-producing substances for years before the carcinogenic nature of these substances becomes evident. It is generally accepted, however, that the cancer risk posed by exposure to chemical carcinogens is small, except under certain industrial working conditions or as a result of environmental industrial pollution. Chemicals released into the

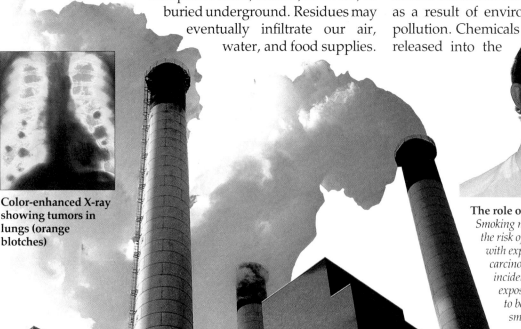

Color-enhanced X-ray showing tumors in lungs (orange blotches)

The role of cigarette smoking
Smoking may significantly increase the risk of cancer when combined with exposure to certain other carcinogens. For example, the incidence of cancer among people exposed to asbestos was found to be much higher among smokers than nonsmokers.

CARCINOGENS IN THE WORKPLACE

Research into occupational cancers has identified three major groups of chemical carcinogens, described at right, and the ways in which they enter the body, shown below. The use of some of these substances has now been banned or is strictly regulated. However, some substances may still be responsible for a small percentage of cancers among people who were exposed in the past or workers who are currently inadequately protected.

Inhalation
The airborne particles, fumes, or by-products of certain substances may lead to cancers of the lungs, larynx, nasal passages, and the covering membranes inside the chest and abdomen.

Ingestion
Certain chemicals can produce cancers in sites such as the bladder or liver if they are swallowed and pass into the bloodstream.

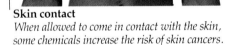

Skin contact
When allowed to come in contact with the skin, some chemicals increase the risk of skin cancers.

AROMATIC AMINES
An aromatic amine, in chemical terms, is any derivative of ammonia that contains one or more benzene rings. There are four aromatic amines known to be carcinogenic to humans.

OCCUPATION	SITE OF CANCER
Dye manufacturers, textile dyers, rubber industry workers, paint makers, coal gas manufacturers, and chemical workers	Bladder

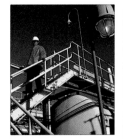

POLYCYCLIC HYDROCARBONS
This group of chemicals is found mainly in tobacco smoke, tar fumes, pitch, solid pitch, soot, tar, and oils.

OCCUPATION	SITE OF CANCER
Asphalt, coal tar, and pitch workers, roofers, coal gas manufacturers, aluminum refiners, welders, miners, and workers exposed to tars and oils	Skin, scrotum, lung, and bladder

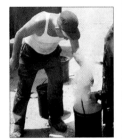

ASBESTOS
Inhaling the airborne particles of asbestos, which is made up of silicate fibers, causes cancer. Three kinds of asbestos were used in the past, each causing a different cancer.

OCCUPATION	SITE OF CANCER
Asbestos miners, asbestos textile manufacturers, insulation workers, shipyard workers, and brake or clutch repairers	Lung, peritoneum, pleura, and larynx

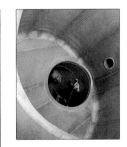

atmosphere are substantially diluted. However, chemical exposure in the workplace presents a greater risk because of the prolonged and sometimes intensive exposure.

OCCUPATIONAL CANCERS

Given the evidence available today, it seems likely that about 4 percent of all fatal cancers in the US are caused by occupational factors. Some of the main groups of carcinogens found in the workplace, and the associated occupations, are listed in the box above. However, there are many other substances used or formed during industrial processes that are also significant carcinogens. For example, benzene – a substance widely used as a solvent in the chemical and drug industries and as a reactant in the synthesis of adhesives and plasters – has been linked to leukemia. Some 2 to 3 million workers may be

**Protecting workers
at risk**
*Our increased knowledge about
the dangers of certain chemicals
has led to improvements in safety
standards in the workplace. People
at risk from exposure to toxic or
carcinogenic substances are issued
protective clothing and safety
equipment (such as that shown
at right, worn by workers
handling chemical wastes).
Unfortunately, safety
precautions are not
adequate in all
countries of the world
(or in all places in the
US) and workers
sometimes ignore
regulations.*

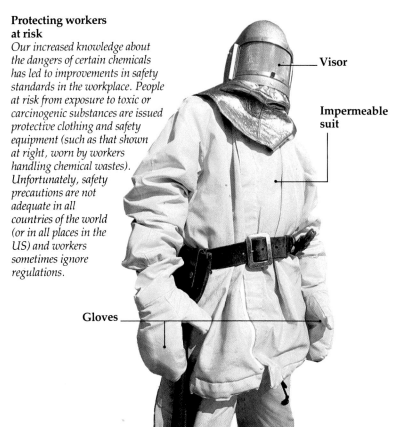

Visor

Impermeable
suit

Gloves

adequate safety precautions are taken to prevent exposure or to limit it to a safe level. Many industries perform regular medical screening of their employees to detect early signs of disease. The screening of people exposed to known carcinogens in the past must be carried out throughout life; some cancers can take 30 years or more to develop.

Any new chemical to which workers are likely to be exposed either at the workplace or at home must be tested for its cancer-causing potential (see TESTS TO IDENTIFY CARCINOGENS below). Testing on animals is performed less often today.

In spite of these improvements, it is likely that some workers are still at risk and a number of occupations (such as rubber, dye, and furniture manufacturing, asbestos fabricating and mining, and nickel refining) are associated with higher-than-normal incidences of cancer. Anyone who works in occupations where there are known risks should observe all recommended precautions.

exposed to benzene in petrochemical, rubber, and coke plants; shoe manufacturers, furniture finishers, and gas station attendants are also exposed to it.

Chromium and its compounds, including chromate salts, are widely used in industries ranging from the manufacture of stainless steel, bricks, and ceramics to the production of paints and dyes. An increased risk of lung cancer has been noted among workers exposed to high levels of chromium and chromates. Additionally, malignant tumors have developed in the livers of workers in polyvinyl chloride factories. Exposure has now been minimized by ventilation in the workplace.

Reducing the risks

Many steps have been taken to improve safety standards in the workplace. The use of many known chemical carcinogens is now prohibited and others are used only if considered essential and if

TESTS TO IDENTIFY CARCINOGENS

A variety of tests exist to detect substances likely to cause cancer in humans. Animals may be injected or exposed to different levels of a suspected carcinogen throughout their life and then examined for signs of tumor development. Today, the most commonly used tests involve the application of suspected carcinogens to isolated cultures of bacterial or mammalian cells to see whether any change occurs in the DNA structure of the cells. Any substance capable of producing such a change is known as a mutagen. While not all carcinogens are mutagenic, such tests have proved remarkably efficient in identifying carcinogens and

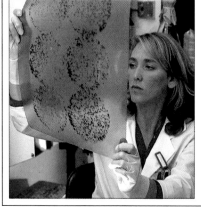

they produce results far more quickly than animal tests.

**Testing for
carcinogens**
*This cancer researcher is
examining a radiation-
sensitive film that has
been exposed to cultures
of radioactively labeled
microorganisms. Testing
the effects of chemicals on
the growth of bacterial
colonies can help identify
carcinogens.*

CASE HISTORY
AN OCCUPATION-LINKED CANCER

Michael had been urinating frequently and his urine had sometimes been tinged with blood. One day he received a letter from his former workplace, a rubber-processing plant, explaining that exposure to certain chemicals in the industry can cause bladder cancer. Medical screening was offered by the company. Michael, now worried by his symptoms, decided to consult his doctor.

PERSONAL DETAILS
Name Michael Kapra
Age 55
Occupation Factory worker
Family No history of disease.

MEDICAL BACKGROUND
Michael has been in good health for most of his life but has a persistent cough due to smoking.

THE CONSULTATION
Michael describes his symptoms to his doctor and shows him the letter he received from his former employer. Concerned, his doctor refers Michael to a urologist who in turn orders tests on his urine.

THE DIAGNOSIS
The urologist tells Michael that the priority is to find the source of his bleeding. He explains that the bladder can be examined by cystoscopy, a process in which a viewing instrument is passed into the bladder through the penis. Michael agrees that the procedure is warranted and the urologist performs the cystoscopic examination, with the aid of an anesthetic jelly, in the office. The procedure reveals a small tumor on the bladder lining. Examination of a small piece of the tumor confirms a diagnosis of BLADDER CANCER. Fortunately, the tumor seems to be at an early stage of development.

THE TREATMENT
The bladder tumor is destroyed by electric cautery through a cystoscope. As an additional precaution, a solution of an anticancer drug is passed into Michael's bladder by catheter each week for about 6 weeks. Michael also learns that cigarette smoking may increase his risk of another bladder tumor and this encourages him to quit.

THE OUTCOME
In his late 30s, Michael was exposed to a group of chemicals called aromatic amines, which are known to cause bladder cancer in humans. The average latent period between exposure and the development of cancer is about 16 years. Luckily, Michael's tumor was detected early enough for treatment to prove successful. He has had no sign of cancer for 6 years, but continues to see his doctor annually because he is still at risk of a recurrence.

Finding the source of the bleeding
Tests on Michael's urine sample confirm the presence of blood. A small tumor in the bladder lining, as shown below, is eventually found to be the cause.

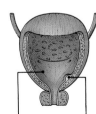

Bladder

Tumor

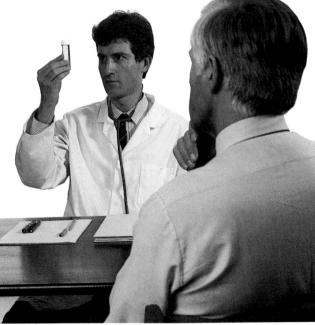

RADIATION, SUNLIGHT, AND CANCER

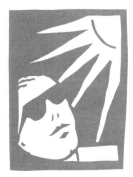

HIGH-ENERGY RADIATION from X-rays, radioactive substances, and cosmic rays penetrates all the cells of the body. Radiation of this ionizing type is a potent cause of cancer. Most people, however, are exposed to only small doses and the risks of getting cancer from these sources are small. There is a much higher risk from the large doses of nonionizing solar radiation that people absorb from excessive sunbathing.

The first case of cancer in a person who worked with X-rays was reported in 1902, within about 7 years of Roentgen's discovery of X-rays. Within 15 years, there were about 100 cases.

It later became apparent that other sources of ionizing radiation (so called because it is capable of displacing electrons from atoms) were equally dangerous. Lung cancer developed in miners working with radioactive uranium ores. And bone cancer often developed in workers who applied radioactive luminous paint to the numerals on the dials of watches and clocks.

Since then, it has been found that ionizing radiation causes an increase in the incidence of almost all types of cancers, and people working with sources of radiation now take the most stringent safeguards to protect themselves. Cancers induced in this way do not appear immediately after exposure but may take as many as 40 years to appear. This, together with the fact that radiation-induced cancers cannot be distinguished from cancers

Sources of ionizing radiation
Most people are exposed to only small doses of ionizing radiation and the risks of cancer from these sources are small – even among people who work with radiation.

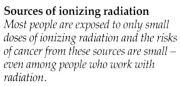
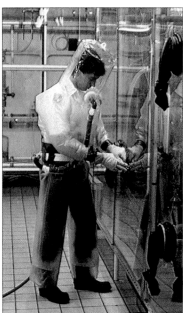
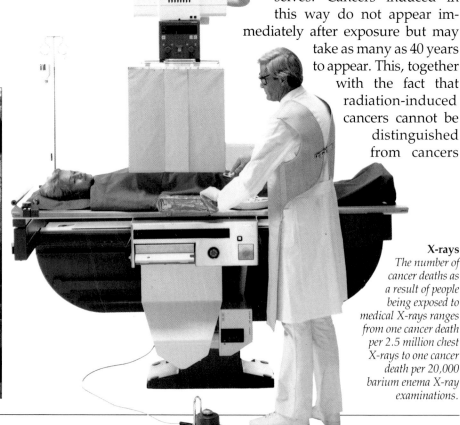

X-rays
The number of cancer deaths as a result of people being exposed to medical X-rays ranges from one cancer death per 2.5 million chest X-rays to one cancer death per 20,000 barium enema X-ray examinations.

caused by any other mechanism, makes it difficult to be certain whether or not a particular tumor occurred spontaneously or was induced by radiation.

HOW RADIATION AFFECTS THE BODY

Ionizing radiation penetrates all the cells of the body, but there is great variation in susceptibility among different cells. Some tissues, such as those of the skeleton, skin, and pancreas, are much less sensitive to radiation than other tissues, such as those of the bone marrow or the lining of the small intestine. Cancer is most likely to occur in tissues that have been directly exposed to radiation, though it can also occur in tissues that have been indirectly exposed.

Dosage
The amount of energy transferred to a particular mass of tissue by radiation is measured in grays. A gray (abbreviated Gy) is a unit of absorbed radiation dose equal to 100 rads.

People who receive doses of radiation greater than 10 grays as a result of accidents at nuclear power plants or from the explosion of nuclear weapons die within 30 days. Doses of 1 to 2 grays will severely damage chromosomes. Smaller doses cause damage that may be delayed for many years.

Even doses of radiation as small as one thousandth of a gray (a milligray) can increase cancer risk in especially susceptible subjects – notably fetuses.

The risks
The only people at high risk of cancer from radiation exposure are those who were within the vicinity of a nuclear explosion (such as occurred at Hiroshima and Nagasaki in 1945) or have been affected directly by radioactive fallout after a nuclear test. Studies of the survivors of such episodes have established that, for every 100,000 people exposed to

HOW RADIATION CAUSES CANCER

There are two ways in which radiation can affect the complex DNA molecules that constitute the chromosomes in cells. One way is by breaking up the DNA molecules; the other is by splitting water molecules in the body and producing free radicals. Either way, the effect is to alter the genetic "program" in cells. It seems almost certain that these mutations are the underlying cause of radiation-induced cancer.

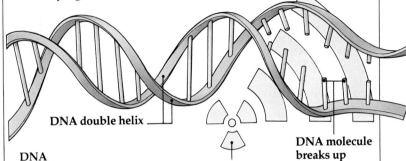

DNA double helix ___

Source of radiation

DNA molecule breaks up

DNA
The atoms that join to form DNA molecules share linking electrons. If these links are knocked out by radiation, the DNA molecules break up, increasing the risk of cancer.

Free radicals
Radiation energy may split water molecules in the body to produce highly active chemical units, called free radicals, which are very damaging to DNA.

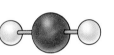

Complete water molecule (H₂O)

Free radical

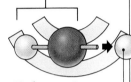

Hydrogen atom breaks away to produce free radical

Vulnerable parts of the body
The cells that undergo constant rapid division and are therefore the most easily damaged by radiation include the cells in the lining of the mouth; the cells in the hair follicles (radiation causes the hair to fall out); the cells in the lining of the intestine (radiation can cause diarrhea); the cells in the bone marrow (radiation can cause anemia); and the germ cells in the testicles and ovaries (radiation can cause sterility).

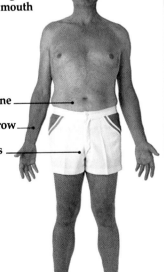

Hair ___

Lining of the mouth

Lining of the intestine ___

Bone marrow ___

Germ cells ___

ASK YOUR DOCTOR
IONIZING AND SOLAR RADIATION

Q My dentist won't give me X-rays while I'm pregnant; she says there is a risk to the fetus. Is she right?

A Yes, she is. Surveys in the US and United Kingdom have established that the children of women who had X-rays during pregnancy have a very small but definitely increased risk of cancer, including leukemia and solid tumors. It is estimated that, for every million fetuses exposed to 10 milligrays of radiation, the radiation may cause as many as 250 fatal cases of cancer during the first 10 years of life. The risk is proportional to the dose, to the number of X-rays given, and to the stage of pregnancy. Radiation in the first three months of pregnancy is five times more likely to cause cancer than radiation in the second or third trimester. Ultrasound examinations have not been shown to carry a risk.

Q Does my regular use of tanning salons increase my risk of skin cancer?

A Tanning salons pose a risk because they increase your exposure to ultraviolet light – the same hazard present in sunlight. If you work in the sun or sunbathe regularly and also visit a tanning salon, you increase your risk of skin cancer significantly.

Q Is a high level of exposure to sunlight particularly dangerous for young children?

A Yes. Melanoma is much less common in the very young, but young children who are exposed to a lot of sun are at risk of melanoma later in life, particularly if they have had recurrent sunburn in childhood.

THE SOURCES OF RADIATION
People receive ionizing radiation in many different ways.

 About 65 percent comes from natural sources, such as rocks, soil, air, and cosmic radiation.

 About 30 percent comes from medical procedures, such as X-rays, radiation therapy, and radioisotopes.

 About 4 percent comes from fallout from nuclear bomb tests.

 Only 1 percent comes from all other sources, including nuclear power and industry.

1 gray of ionizing radiation, approximately 1,250 will die of radiation-induced cancers. We have yet to learn the effect of radiation on those involved at, or within the vicinity of, the Chernobyl nuclear power plant accident that occurred in the USSR in 1986.

In contrast, the level of radiation to which the average person is exposed from natural sources (e.g., radiation from rocks, from radioactive gases such as radon released from rocks, and from cosmic rays) is thought to produce only about four fatal cancers a year in each 100,000 people.

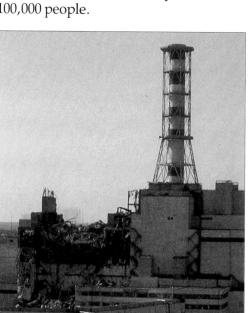

Nuclear accident
People involved in an accident at a nuclear plant, such as the one that occurred in Chernobyl in the USSR in 1986, are at high risk of cancer from radiation exposure, though such cancers may take up to 40 years to develop.

OCCUPATIONAL RADIATION

People who work with radiation receive an average dose of 4 milligrays (4 thousandths of a gray) per year, which would be expected to cause 50 cancer deaths per million workers. By comparison, the annual death rate from accidents per million construction workers is about 200; per million coal miners, about 250; and per million deep sea fishermen, about 2,500. Recent research in the United Kingdom has, however, suggested that exposure of male workers to radiation in nuclear plants can lead to damage to sperm cells and to a small but increased risk of leukemia in their children.

In most cases, there is probably nothing a person can do to reduce his or her risk of radiation-induced cancer. The cancers that can possibly be avoided are those from exposure to unnecessary X-rays and those that occur in people who work with radiation.

THE SUN AND SKIN CANCER

Skin cancer ranks high among the avoidable cancers related to life-style. It is avoidable because most people have some choice in the amount of exposure to sunlight they receive.

The damaging feature of sunlight is the ultraviolet B component. The amount of ultraviolet B an individual absorbs depends on factors such as distance from the equator, altitude, sky cover, and time of day and year. The greatest amount occurs during the summer months, and about a third of the day's total amount occurs between the hours of 11 AM and 1 PM.

Another factor that affects exposure to ultraviolet B is ozone in the atmosphere. Ozone absorbs most of the ultraviolet

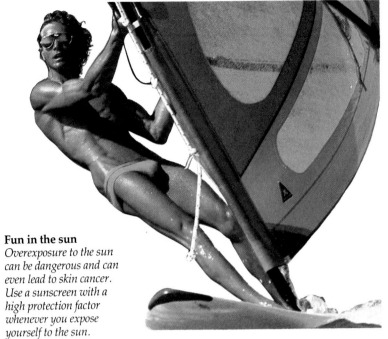

Fun in the sun
Overexposure to the sun can be dangerous and can even lead to skin cancer. Use a sunscreen with a high protection factor whenever you expose yourself to the sun.

light in the upper stratosphere and allows only small amounts to reach the earth. There is growing concern today about the damage to the ozone layer being caused by a variety of gases released on Earth.

Nonmelanoma skin cancer
Basal cell carcinoma, the most common kind of skin cancer in light-skinned people, usually affects the face and neck. Early removal cures it. The same applies to squamous cell carcinoma, the second most common type of skin cancer. If not treated, both cancers can cause severe and extensive tissue destruction and may even be fatal.

Melanoma
Excessive exposure to sunlight can also increase the risk of malignant melanoma, which is much rarer but far more dangerous and causes a substantial number of deaths. Melanoma can also occur in individuals who do not spend time in the sun. A change in a mole, for example, can occur with or without sun exposure. As with other forms of skin cancer, early detection and treatment of melanoma is vital.

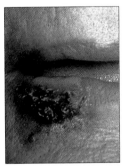

Nonmelanoma skin cancer
Its occurrence is strongly linked to exposure to sunlight.

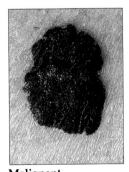

Malignant melanoma
Australians have a high rate of melanoma. However, they have learned the warning signs of cancer and get treatment early.

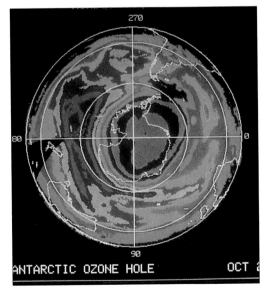

270

80

0

90

ANTARCTIC OZONE HOLE   OCT

The ozone layer
Satellite photographs reveal areas of thinning, or even "holes," in the Earth's ozone layer. The blue area in the center of the photograph above corresponds to one such hole over Antarctica.

VIRUSES AND CANCER

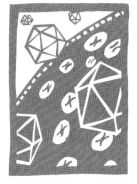

VIRUSES ARE RELATIVELY simple life-forms that cause a wide range of disease in humans – from influenza and rabies to warts and cold sores. Viruses cause disease by entering body cells to replicate. In doing so, they may seriously interfere with the function of (and may ultimately kill) the host cells. Several types of viruses have been linked to human cancers.

A virus particle consists of some genetic material enclosed in one or two shells, or capsules. Many viruses have the ability to incorporate their own genetic material into the genetic material (DNA) of their host cells, which alters the DNA of the host cells. This is the type of change in cells that researchers believe activates or deactivates oncogenes (cancer-causing genes) and turns normal cells into cancerous cells. There is thus an obvious mechanism by which viruses might cause cancer.

CANCERS LINKED TO VIRUSES

In practice, just five cancers have been associated with a viral cause – cervical cancer, liver cancer, penile cancer, Burkitt's lymphoma, and T-cell leukemia. Of these, only cervical cancer is common in the US. The human immunodeficiency virus (HIV), the AIDS virus, increases susceptibility to several types of cancer through its effect on the immune system.

What are viruses?
Viruses are the smallest known infectious agents, measuring between one millionth and one hundred thousandth of an inch in diameter. Most of them cannot be seen even with a powerful light microscope. The number of different viruses probably exceeds the number of all other organisms. The diseases caused by viruses range from the harmless, such as the common cold, to extremely serious and life-threatening diseases, such as AIDS. Viruses have only a few variants in their basic structure, but come in various shapes and sizes.

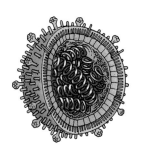

Human immunodeficiency virus (HIV)

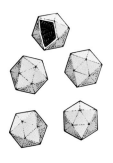

Papillomavirus (wart virus)

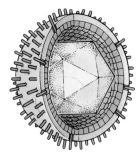

Epstein-Barr virus

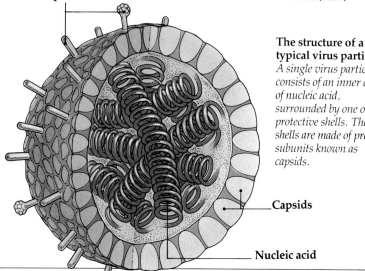

Surface proteins

The structure of a typical virus particle
A single virus particle consists of an inner core of nucleic acid, surrounded by one or two protective shells. The shells are made of protein subunits known as capsids.

Capsids

Nucleic acid

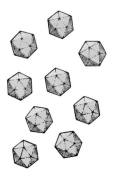

Hepatitis virus B

Human T-cell lymphotropic virus (HTLV-I)

HOW VIRUSES CAUSE DISEASE

The sole activity of viruses is to invade the cells of other organisms, which they take over to make copies of themselves. Certain viruses may, in the process of replication, modify the genetic material contained within the chromosomes of the host cell and prompt the cell and its successors to become cancerous.

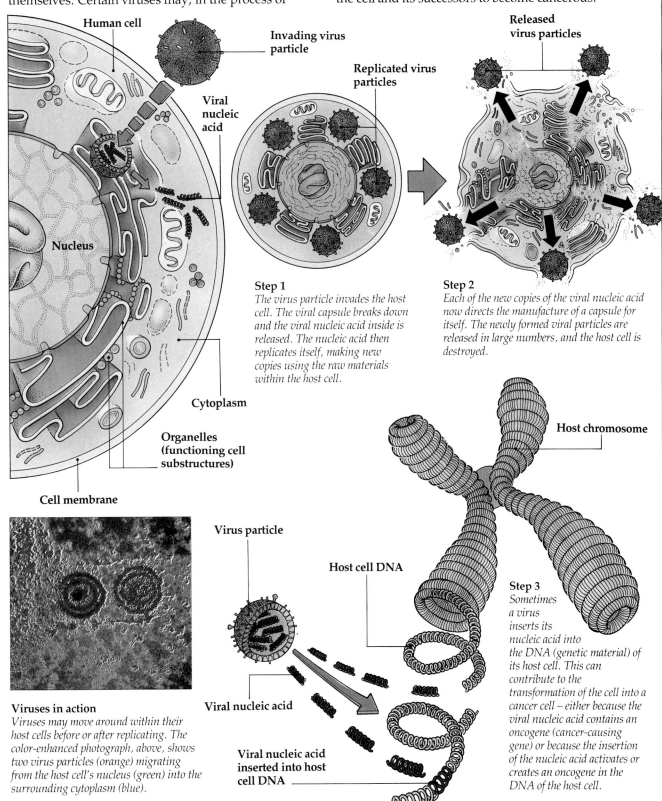

Human cell

Invading virus particle

Viral nucleic acid

Replicated virus particles

Released virus particles

Nucleus

Cytoplasm

Organelles (functioning cell substructures)

Cell membrane

Step 1
The virus particle invades the host cell. The viral capsule breaks down and the viral nucleic acid inside is released. The nucleic acid then replicates itself, making new copies using the raw materials within the host cell.

Step 2
Each of the new copies of the viral nucleic acid now directs the manufacture of a capsule for itself. The newly formed viral particles are released in large numbers, and the host cell is destroyed.

Host chromosome

Virus particle

Host cell DNA

Viral nucleic acid

Viral nucleic acid inserted into host cell DNA

Step 3
Sometimes a virus inserts its nucleic acid into the DNA (genetic material) of its host cell. This can contribute to the transformation of the cell into a cancer cell – either because the viral nucleic acid contains an oncogene (cancer-causing gene) or because the insertion of the nucleic acid activates or creates an oncogene in the DNA of the host cell.

Viruses in action
Viruses may move around within their host cells before or after replicating. The color-enhanced photograph, above, shows two virus particles (orange) migrating from the host cell's nucleus (green) into the surrounding cytoplasm (blue).

Cervical cancer

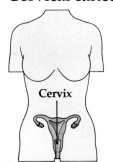

Cervix

Cervical cancer occurs almost exclusively in women who have had sexual intercourse. The risk of cervical cancer increases with an early onset of sexual activity and with the number of sexual partners a woman has had (and her partners have had). This evidence suggests that a virus, passed from men to women during sexual intercourse, is involved in causing cervical cancer. At one time, the virus responsible for genital herpes (herpes simplex II virus) was suspected. However, human papillomavirus, or the wart virus, is now considered a much stronger contender. There are scores of wart viruses and only some types are thought to cause cancer. Other factors, including smoking and possibly herpes virus infection, may work together with wart virus infection to cause cervical cancer.

Liver cancer

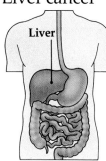

Liver

Primary liver cancer is very strongly associated with hepatitis virus B infection and now has also been related to hepatitis virus C. In some parts of Africa and Asia, as many as 30 percent of the people are carriers of hepatitis virus B (the carrier rate in the US is only 0.1 percent), and in those areas the prevalence of primary liver cancer is extremely high. Long-standing carriers of hepatitis virus B are 200 times as likely to have liver cancer as noncarriers. The exact role played by hepatitis viruses in liver cancer is not clear, however. Primary liver cancer does occur in people who are not infected with hepatitis B or C viruses, and most carriers of those viruses do not get cancer.

HOW VIRAL HEPATITIS TYPE B IS SPREAD

Hepatitis virus B is spread in precisely the same ways as the human immunodeficiency virus (HIV), the virus responsible for AIDS.

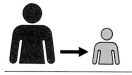

In newborns
Hepatitis virus B can be passed on to a newborn baby if his or her mother is a carrier.

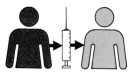

By needle sharing
The virus can be spread by an infected person's blood coming into contact with someone else's – as when needles are shared among drug abusers.

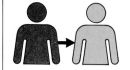

By sexual transmission
The virus can be sexually transmitted by men and women and is particularly common among male homosexuals.

Burkitt's lymphoma

Burkitt's lymphoma is a malignancy of the lymph glands in the jaw. It is rare in the US, mainly affecting children in areas of tropical Africa and New Guinea.

The research done to date suggests that the virus that causes infectious mononucleosis, the Epstein-Barr virus, is also involved in causing Burkitt's lymphoma. For example, cells from Burkitt's lymphoma have bits of genetic material from the Epstein-Barr virus incorporated in their own genetic material.

However, the Epstein-Barr virus is common worldwide, and people in the US who get infectious mononucleosis

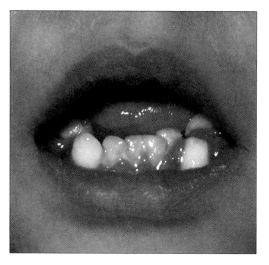

Burkitt's lymphoma
This cancer of the lymph tissues, which is confined almost exclusively to children living in Africa and New Guinea, causes an enlarging tumor or tumors within the jaw and/or the abdomen. The photograph shows a child with a tumor on the left-hand side of the jaw that has displaced several teeth.

do not get Burkitt's lymphoma, so it is likely that other factors are also at work. Because Burkitt's lymphoma occurs in parts of the world where malaria is highly prevalent, it is speculated that malaria in early life alters the body's response to the virus so that, when the Epstein-Barr virus infection occurs, it leads to malignant change.

T-cell leukemia

T-cell leukemia is a very rare leukemia that occurs in only a few parts of the world, including southern Japan and the Caribbean (a few cases have occurred in the US among immigrants from the Caribbean). Like other leukemias, the abnormal cells are found in the blood and bone marrow throughout the body rather than grouped into a tumor. It is now known to be caused by the human T-cell lymphotropic virus (HTLV-I) – a virus closely related to human immuno-deficiency virus (the AIDS virus). HTLV-I infects the cells of the body's immune system known as T cells. It is transmitted by blood transfusion, by sexual activity, and to infants at birth. The virus was discovered in the early 1980s.

Kaposi's sarcoma

Kaposi's sarcoma is a type of malignant tumor of the skin, intestines, lymph glands, and other tissues. This cancer used to be very rare, occurring for un-known reasons in older men. Today in the US, Kaposi's sarcoma occurs almost exclusively in people who have AIDS.

The human immunodeficiency virus (the AIDS virus) interferes with the cells of the body's immune system called T cells. T cells are known to be responsible, among other things, for "immunological surveillance" of cancer cells, helping the body to get rid of cells that might other-wise develop into cancers. Doctors therefore presume that Kaposi's sarco-ma, as well as other cancers, occurs in people whose T cells have lost their im-munological surveillance function.

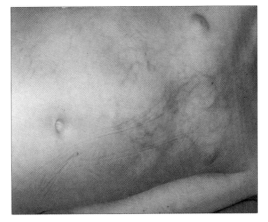

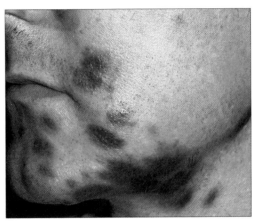

T-cell leukemia
This is a rare form of leukemia, caused by a virus, that infects the cells of the body's immune system known as T cells. The prominent veins in the patient shown are caused by enlarged lymph glands pressing on the superior vena cava (a large vein in the chest) and causing pressure within the veins of the upper part of the body.

Kaposi's sarcoma
One of the manifestations of Kaposi's sarcoma is the appearance of malignant skin tumors consisting of purple-red patches, which usually start on the feet and ankles, spread up the legs, and then appear on the hands and arms.

OUTLOOK

Only recently has the ability of a virus to cause cancer been confirmed. However, there are other factors to consider. First, most of the viruses that have been associ-ated with cancer do not cause cancer by themselves; they usually require another cancer-causing agent before they can ex-ert this effect. Second, many viruses are transmitted from one person to another by methods that are controllable. For example, the sexual transmission of wart viruses can be prevented by seeking treatment and by using condoms. Third, the discovery that a virus is the cause of a cancer opens up the possibility that the cancer can be fought by devising strate-gies against the virus – through the de-velopment and use of new vaccines. There is hope that the incidence of liver cancer throughout the world can be lessened by using hepatitis B vaccines.

SEX, DRUGS, REPRODUCTION, AND CANCER

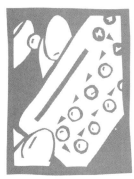

I N ADDITION TO THE BETTER-KNOWN FACTORS that can affect cancer risk – such as smoking – there are several other variables that can increase or decrease your risk of cancer. These include taking certain types of drugs and hormones (including oral contraceptives), your sexual behavior, your reproductive history, and whether or not you have been circumcised.

Drug treatment is believed to play a part in less than 1 percent of cancers. Your sexual behavior and reproductive history can, however, significantly affect your cancer risk, especially the risk of cancers associated with AIDS and cancers of the female reproductive organs.

DRUGS AND CANCER

Only a small number of drugs have been implicated as causing cancer. Most drugs known to pose a cancer risk (even for animals) never reach the market.

HORMONES, PREGNANCY, AND CANCER

The effect of certain hormone-based drugs and of pregnancy on the chances of acquiring certain cancers is summarized below.

Ovarian cancer
Use of oral contraceptives may decrease the risk of this cancer.

Having a child in early adulthood also appears to decrease the risk.

Vaginal and cervical cancer
Diethylstilbestrol (DES) was prescribed in the 1940s and 1950s to prevent pregnant women from having miscarriages. Women who were exposed, before birth, to DES were later found to be at significantly increased risk of certain rare types of vaginal and cervical cancer. As a result, doctors stopped prescribing DES for the prevention of miscarriage in the late 1970s.

Some studies have shown a weak link between use of oral contraceptives and an increased risk of cervical cancer.

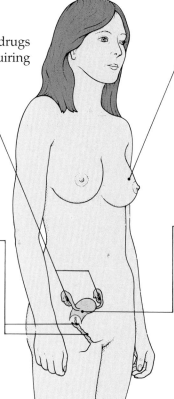

Breast cancer
Some studies have shown that taking oral contraceptives slightly increases the risk of breast cancer; other studies have shown no link.

Having a child in early adulthood seems to be a protective factor. Women whose first pregnancy occurs later in life or who do not have children appear to be at a slightly increased risk.

Cancer of the endometrium (lining of the uterus)
Use of oral contraceptives may decrease the risk of this cancer.

Having a child early in adulthood appears to be a protective factor.

Having hormone replacement therapy with estrogens only after the menopause was found to increase the risk of endometrial cancer. Today, such therapy has been modified by adding a progestogen to the estrogen. This treatment is thought to make hormone replacement therapy much safer.

Hormone-based drugs

The effects of hormone-based drugs (including oral contraceptives and hormone replacement therapy) on the risk of cancers that occur in women are summarized in the box on HORMONES, PREGNANCY, AND CANCER on page 60.

Immunosuppressive drugs

The body's immune system plays an important role in the prevention of cancer. Immunosuppressive drugs reduce the efficiency of the immune system and can lead to an increased risk of cancer. This risk is considered acceptable when drugs are given to organ transplant patients to help them accept a "foreign" organ.

Anticancer drugs

Anticancer drugs, used in chemotherapy, act by interfering with the multiplication of cancer cells. These drugs are also capable of causing damage that may lead to cancer in normal cells. Although anticancer drugs have prolonged the lives of thousands of cancer patients, they may also have caused cancer in a small number of them.

SEXUAL BEHAVIOR AND REPRODUCTION

Sexual behavior and reproduction can affect cancer risk in a number of ways.

Number of sexual partners

A clear association has been found between the risk of cervical cancer and the number of sexual partners a woman and her partners have had. The risk is also linked to the age at which she first had sexual intercourse. The common denominator is thought to be an infectious agent – probably two or more strains of the papillomavirus (the wart virus).

Human immunodeficiency virus (HIV, the AIDS virus) and hepatitis B virus are both linked with certain cancers. The viruses can be sexually transmitted. The risks of infection can be re-

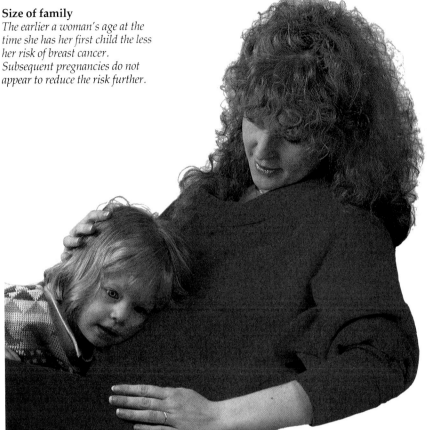

Size of family
The earlier a woman's age at the time she has her first child the less her risk of breast cancer. Subsequent pregnancies do not appear to reduce the risk further.

duced by limiting the number of sexual partners, by exercising caution in choice of partners, and by practicing "safe" sex, including the use of condoms.

Reproduction

The incidence of breast cancer increases with the length of a woman's reproductive life. Women who start menstruating early and who have a late menopause are at a higher risk.

Women who have their first child early are at decreased risk of cancers of the breast, endometrium, and ovary compared to those who have their first child later in life or who do not have children.

A pregnancy that ends in miscarriage or abortion does not appear to have the same protective effect on breast cancer as a pregnancy that goes full-term. It is thought that the beneficial effect of pregnancy is produced by the stimulation to the breasts to form milk that a full-term pregnancy provides.

CIRCUMCISION

Cancer of the penis predominantly affects uncircumcised men who have not practiced scrupulous hygiene, often due to a tight foreskin. Cancer of the penis rarely occurs in men who were circumcised at birth. Uncircumcised men should keep the area under the foreskin clean by washing it daily. There is also some evidence that women who have intercourse only with circumcised men have a lesser chance of getting cancer of the cervix than women whose partners are uncircumcised.

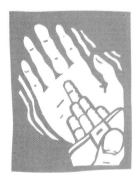

THE ANTICANCER LIFE-STYLE

SOME CANCERS, SUCH AS TUMORS of the brain and spinal cord, occur for reasons that are little understood, and so it is not known how they can be prevented. However, for many of the more common cancers, researchers have identified specific causes. Today, each of us has the opportunity to reduce his or her cancer risk by following the recommendations of the "anticancer life-style."

Too many people who are educated about the risks of cancer make little alteration in their life-styles. Consequently, thousands of cancers occur that might easily have been prevented.

CANCER PREVENTION

To reduce your chances of getting cancer, follow these two forms of preventive activity. First, avoid or minimize exposure to known carcinogenic agents, such as tobacco and tobacco smoke, alcohol, and excess ultraviolet radiation from the sun and tanning devices. Second, monitor your body for the warning signs of cancer, take prompt action if you find any of the recognized signs or symptoms, and undergo recommended medical screening procedures, such as cervical (Pap) smears (see Chapter Four on SYMPTOMS, SCREENING, AND DIAGNOSIS).

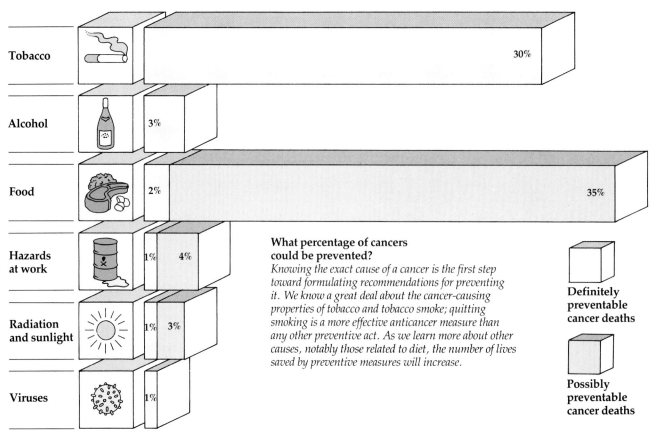

Tobacco 30%

Alcohol 3%

Food 2% 35%

Hazards at work 1% 4%

Radiation and sunlight 1% 3%

Viruses 1%

What percentage of cancers could be prevented?
Knowing the exact cause of a cancer is the first step toward formulating recommendations for preventing it. We know a great deal about the cancer-causing properties of tobacco and tobacco smoke; quitting smoking is a more effective anticancer measure than any other preventive act. As we learn more about other causes, notably those related to diet, the number of lives saved by preventive measures will increase.

Definitely preventable cancer deaths

Possibly preventable cancer deaths

CHECKLIST FOR THE ANTICANCER LIFE-STYLE

The changes in cell structure that can lead to cancer occur in many different parts of the body. For this reason, the principles of primary cancer prevention must take into account recommendations that affect a wide range of life-style factors.

Tobacco use

Inhaling tobacco smoke carries more risk of cancer than any other activity. Noninhaling smokers are also at risk of mouth, throat, and esophageal cancers. Using smokeless forms of tobacco, such as snuff or chewing tobacco, also causes cancer. Quitting smoking, or never starting, is by far the most important single anticancer measure.

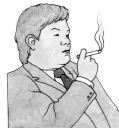

Sunlight

To reduce the risk of skin cancer, fair-skinned people, especially those who sunbathe, should limit their exposure to the sun and use a sunscreen with a high protection factor. To further reduce your risk of skin cancer, avoid using sunlamps and tanning salons.

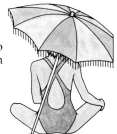

Diet

The National Cancer Institute has published anticancer recommendations affecting several aspects of diet (see DIETARY RECOMMENDATIONS on page 41). Reducing dietary fat, increasing fiber, including a variety of vegetables and fruits in the daily diet, and not eating or eating sparingly smoked, nitrate-cured, and salted foods improve your chances of avoiding cancer.

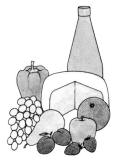

Sexual practices

Cancer of the cervix is more common in women who have multiple partners and whose partners have multiple partners. Good hygiene, attention to warning symptoms, the use of condoms, and the choice of fewer partners all reduce the risk. Circumcision also reduces the risk of cancer of the penis, which usually starts inside the foreskin.

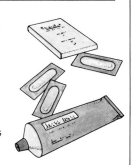

Obesity

If your weight exceeds the upper limit of the ideal weight range for your height and build by more than 20 percent, you have an increased risk of cancer. Maintaining your body weight within the ideal range for your size gives valuable protection against cancer.

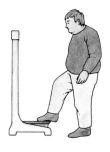

Viruses

Certain viruses, including the viruses that cause hepatitis B and C and venereal warts, as well as the AIDS virus, are linked to cancer. Prevention of virus-linked cancer involves minimizing exposure to the viruses responsible, many of which are transmitted sexually.

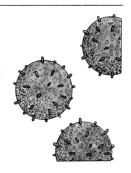

Alcohol

Excessive alcohol intake is associated with increased risk of several types of cancer, especially when taken in conjunction with tobacco. Alcoholic drinks also have a high calorie content and therefore carry a secondary cancer risk in that their calories can contribute to obesity in sedentary people.

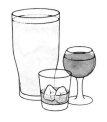

Drugs

People who are prescribed synthetic "replacement" estrogens, immuno-suppressive agents, and some anticancer drugs should discuss with their doctors whether the need justifies the use of these medications, which increase their risk of cancer.

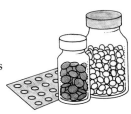

Radiation

Anyone undergoing extensive medical treatment involving multiple X-rays should be aware that the radiation could be harmful. Any woman who believes she could be pregnant should tell her doctor before being X-rayed.

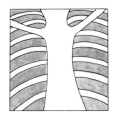

Occupations

All workers in industry and manufacturing should be aware of potentially cancer-causing substances in the workplace and should observe all recommended precautions to avoid or reduce exposure.

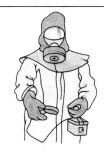

CHAPTER FOUR

SYMPTOMS, SCREENING, AND DIAGNOSIS

DESPITE TAKING ALL known measures to reduce the risks, a cancer may develop at some time in a person's life through factors beyond his or her control. Given this fact, the importance of early diagnosis can hardly be overemphasized. Cancer always starts with a very small cell mass and then grows. In general, the seriousness of a cancer is related to its size. Cancer that is confined to the site of origin is often curable; but a cancer that has already spread to other parts of the body is always very serious. Not so many years ago, cancer that had metastasized (spread) was considered incurable and in most cases was not even treated. Today, the situation is improved; some cancers are curable even in an advanced stage. However, the distinction between localized and metastasized cancer is an essential one. In general, a localized cancer is more responsive to treatment and likely to be curable. Early diagnosis is necessary to maximize the chances of recovery and to minimize chemotherapy, which carries risks of toxicity. Any measure that promotes early diagnosis is of vital importance.

The first section of this chapter, SYMPTOMS OF CANCER, discusses the warning symptoms that should be brought to the attention of your doctor as soon as they occur. Cancer is by no means the only diagnosis that could be concluded from the symptoms mentioned. However, this is no reason for delaying a medical examination. The alternative diagnoses may be equally serious. It is comforting to realize, however, that most symptoms that we associate with cancer do not necessarily signal cancer. This section also discusses methods of self-examination that may help you detect cancer, particularly breast, testicular, and skin cancers.

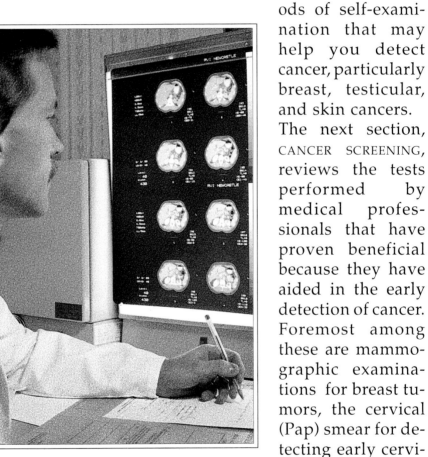

The next section, CANCER SCREENING, reviews the tests performed by medical professionals that have proven beneficial because they have aided in the early detection of cancer. Foremost among these are mammographic examinations for breast tumors, the cervical (Pap) smear for detecting early cervical cancer, and tests for colorectal cancer. The final section, DIAGNOSIS AND ASSESSMENT, explains the procedures commonly performed in reaching a diagnosis of cancer, including special tests such as endoscopy, imaging techniques, and biopsy procedures. The concept of staging a cancer – assessing how far it has developed and spread before treatment options are considered – is also explained.

SYMPTOMS OF CANCER

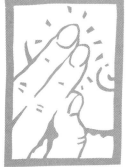

N O ONE WOULD SUGGEST that cancer can always be avoided. However, we can reduce the risks. Cancer will develop in about one in four of us. For this reason, it is important that everyone be sensitive to the earliest indications of cancer so that treatment can be obtained before too much damage is done or the cancer has progressed to an inoperable or untreatable stage.

SEVEN MAJOR WARNING SIGNS OF CANCER

Because you are the person who is most familiar with your body, you are in the best position to detect any abnormal changes. This is why regular self-examination is an important means of detecting cancer. Most breast cancers are discovered by patients, not by doctors.

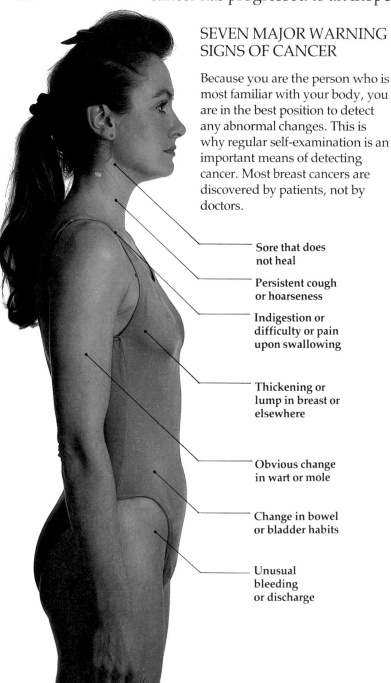

Sore that does not heal

Persistent cough or hoarseness

Indigestion or difficulty or pain upon swallowing

Thickening or lump in breast or elsewhere

Obvious change in wart or mole

Change in bowel or bladder habits

Unusual bleeding or discharge

When cancer develops, an ongoing change begins in the body. Each of us should be aware of the manifestations of such a change. This section alerts you to warning symptoms and signs and describes the methods you can use to examine yourself to increase your chances of detecting cancer early.

WHAT ARE THE SYMPTOMS OF CANCER?

Most cancers signal their presence at an early stage when complete cure is often possible. However, it is not always easy to recognize the very early symptoms of cancer because sometimes they are vague. For instance, feeling under the weather or having a slight fever for one day shouldn't worry you. However, you should take these symptoms seriously if they persist.

There are also more specific signs and symptoms that may occur in the early stages of cancer. The American Cancer Society has compiled a list summarizing the principal warning signs of cancer (see illustration at left). If you notice any of these symptoms you should contact your doctor immediately. These warning signs, along with some additional signs that could signal trouble, are discussed in more detail in the sections that follow. The more obvious signs are discussed under SYMPTOMS TO TAKE SERIOUSLY on page 69. The signs that would probably come to your attention only during close visual inspection or by touch are covered in the illustrated self-examination boxes

MONITOR YOUR SYMPTOMS
LOSS OF APPETITE

Many middle-aged and elderly people suffering from a persistent loss of appetite automatically assume that they may have cancer. But many other disorders are more commonly responsible for loss of appetite in these age groups. Most of these are serious, but treatable. However, a doctor should always be consulted if anyone of any age does not regain his or her appetite.

LOSS OF APPETITE IN CHILDREN

You should consult your doctor if your child suddenly loses his or her appetite and eats little or nothing for more than 24 hours. Such symptoms are usually due to infections (cancer is rare in childhood).

BEGIN HERE

Appetite loss accompanied by persistent changes in bowel habit, nausea, vomiting, or blood in the stool may indicate that you have a serious digestive tract disorder. *Have you had any of these symptoms?*

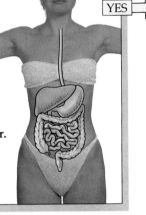

YES →

CONSULT YOUR DOCTOR WITHOUT DELAY!

Ulceration, inflammation, or possibly cancer of the gastrointestinal tract could be causing your symptoms.

Action The doctor will discuss your medical history and you will probably have a thorough physical examination. The doctor will then determine if any additional testing is necessary.

Psychological illness can sometimes cause a lack of interest in food.
Have you had one or more of the following symptoms?
◆ *Apathy*
◆ *Difficulty sleeping*
◆ *Inability to concentrate*
◆ *Loss of interest in sex*

NO

↓

A sudden loss of appetite accompanied by profuse night sweats could be a sign of a lung infection or other infections. *Have you had any of the following symptoms?*
◆ *Raised temperature*
◆ *Persistent cough*
◆ *Blood-stained phlegm*

NO →

Appetite loss accompanied by night sweats and swollen glands in the neck, armpits, or groin may mean that you have a chronic infection or cancer of the lymph glands. *Have you noticed these symptoms?*

NO

NO   **YES**

↓

Depression is one of several problems (such as anxiety) that could cause your symptoms.

Action Consult your doctor. If he or she suspects the cause of your symptoms is psychological, you may be referred to a specialist.

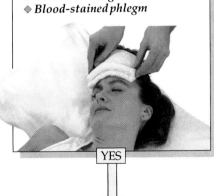

YES

↓

Tuberculosis, another infection, or lung cancer is a possibility.

Action Consult your doctor, who will examine you and may order a chest X-ray and take samples of blood and phlegm.

YES

↓

CONSULT YOUR DOCTOR WITHOUT DELAY!

An infection (such as toxoplasmosis), Hodgkin's disease (lymph gland cancer), other cancers, or a chronic infection may be the cause.

Action After a careful taking of your medical history and a physical examination, your doctor will determine the appropriate tests.

Action Talk to your doctor if you are unable to make a diagnosis from the information given here.

MONITOR YOUR SYMPTOMS
UNUSUAL BUMPS AND LUMPS

An unexplained lump or swelling on any part of the body is one of the most significant signs of cancer. Fortunately, the vast majority of such lumps are not malignant. Most are a sign of infection or allergy or are benign tumors or cysts and can, in most cases, be successfully and easily treated. However, because cancer is a possibility, you should always consult your doctor if you find any new lumps.

> **LUMPS IN CHILDREN**
> Swollen glands commonly develop in children under 10 years old who have minor infections such as a cold. This is no cause for concern. If, however, your child has one or more persistent, painless lumps or swellings underneath the skin, you should consult your doctor.

BEGIN HERE

Is the lump in your breast?

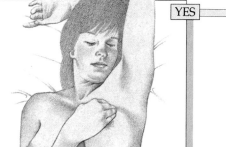

YES

CONSULT YOUR DOCTOR WITHOUT DELAY!

Any lump in the breast should be examined by a doctor to eliminate the chance of breast cancer, even though other harmless causes, such as a benign tumor or a cyst, are more likely.

Action After examining your breasts, if the doctor thinks there is any cause for concern, he or she will arrange for you to have a mammogram and a biopsy.

NO

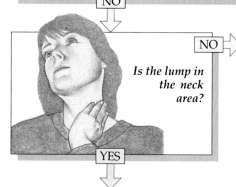

Is the lump in the neck area?

NO

Do you have a lump in the upper part of your abdomen?

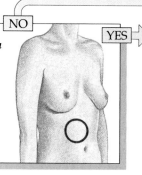

NO

YES

Such a lump could be an aneurysm (pulsating swelling) of the large blood vessel (the aorta) or a swollen liver resulting from heart failure, lymphoma (lymph gland cancer), or cancer.
Does the lump expand with each heartbeat?

YES

NO

YES

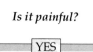

Is it painful?

NO

CONSULT YOUR DOCTOR WITHOUT DELAY!

A salivary gland disorder may be present or a cancer in the throat is a possibility.

Action If cancer is suspected, a small sample of tissue will be taken for microscope examination and your larynx, throat, lungs, and esophagus will be examined through a viewing tube.

An aortic aneurysm is a possibility.

Action Consult your doctor right away. If, after examining you, the doctor suspects an aneurysm, you will be referred to the hospital for tests, such as ultrasound and angiography.

YES

Painful swellings along with a sore throat may be due to tonsillitis, another low-grade infection, or to infectious mononucleosis. See your doctor.
Do you also have swellings in the armpit or groin?

YES

NO

Tonsillitis or another mouth or throat infection is the most likely diagnosis.

Action Symptoms may be relieved by painkillers; smoking and drinking should be avoided. Consult your doctor if symptoms continue for more than 48 hours.

Infectious mononucleosis or another viral infection may be the explanation for your symptoms.

Action Consult your doctor who, after performing an examination, will arrange for you to have a blood test. Your doctor may also perform other tests to rule out cancer of the lymph glands.

Have you noticed a small, pale lump in the skin? **YES** ➤

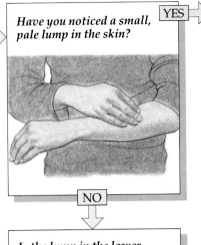

NO

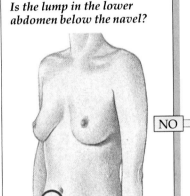

Is the lump in the lower abdomen below the navel?

YES

NO ◄

CONSULT YOUR DOCTOR WITHOUT DELAY!

Most skin swellings are benign but skin cancer is a possibility.

Action Diagnosis of skin cancer is based on microscope examination of a sample of tissue.

Action Talk to your doctor if you have any more questions.

NO

Is the lump a swollen testicle?

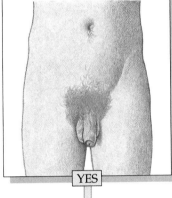

YES

Any benign or malignant enlargement of the organs in the lower abdomen or pelvis may be responsible (such as cancer of the ovary or bladder).

Action Consult your doctor who will perform a thorough examination. An examination with a viewing tube may be performed to look for the cause.

CONSULT YOUR DOCTOR WITHOUT DELAY!

Heart failure, lymphoma, or cancer that has spread to the liver or other organs in the abdomen could be causing your symptoms.

Action The doctor will perform a physical examination and may perform a variety of other tests. If lymphoma or another cancer is suspected, a biopsy will be taken.

CONSULT YOUR DOCTOR WITHOUT DELAY!

A cyst is the most common cause of a swollen testicle but cancer of the testicle is also a possibility.

Action The doctor will examine both testicles and may arrange for an ultrasound examination of the testicle and for other tests. Cancer can be definitely diagnosed only by removal of the testicle and analysis of the tissue. This procedure is performed only after all other possible diagnoses have been eliminated.

on pages 70, 72, 74, and 75. A few selected signs are detailed in the charts on pages 67, 68, and 73.

The fear factor

The fact that you have any of these signs or symptoms does not necessarily mean that you have cancer. Because cancer is so much less common than the many other conditions that could cause these symptoms, the probability is that the symptoms have another explanation. Even so, never ignore such symptoms. Some people do not report their symptoms to their doctor because they fear that cancer may be the diagnosis, or because they are afraid of the eventual treatment. Some people waste time postponing action because of fear, only to find that they do have cancer but now it has become inoperable. If you give your doctor a clear description of your symptoms, he or she can arrange for tests or an appointment with a specialist. Either decision can help eliminate your fears and lead to early, and often successful, treatment.

SYMPTOMS TO TAKE SERIOUSLY

The following symptoms indicate that cancer is a possibility, and should always be taken seriously. In most cases, a diagnosis other than cancer is likely. For this reason, we list some of the other possible conditions that can cause the same symptoms. Nevertheless, if you have a symptom that represents a change in the way your body functions, consult your doctor.

Unexplained weight loss

Unexplained loss of weight is often a feature of cancer and should lead you to seek the advice of your doctor. However, remember that weight loss can also be caused by other conditions, including chronic infection and depression.

Loss of appetite

See the symptoms chart on page 67.

SKIN SELF-EXAMINATION

The incidence of skin cancer has increased tremendously in the last 10 years. The American Cancer Society recommends that men and women of all ages perform regular skin self-examinations. This is particularly important if you are light-skinned and over 30. Basal cell carcinoma is the most common type of skin cancer, followed by squamous cell carcinoma. Once diagnosed, the majority of these cancers are easily treated. The rarest and most serious type of skin cancer is malignant melanoma. Perform your examination in a well-lighted room, preferably in front of a full-length mirror. You also will need a small hand mirror and may want to use a magnifying glass.

WHAT TO LOOK FOR

◆ A change in color or toughening, thickening, or puckering of the skin.
◆ A sore that fails to heal within 3 weeks.
◆ A mole or blemish that changes shape or color, itches, or bleeds.

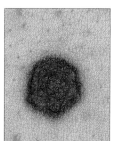

Normal mole
A common mole is almost symmetrical, clearly delineated from surrounding skin, flat or evenly elevated, and usually tan to dark brown and evenly pigmented.

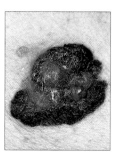

Malignant melanoma
Use the ABCD test to check for the following danger signs.
Asymmetry
Border – irregular or unclear
Color – very dark brown, blue, or black
Diameter – greater than ¼ inch

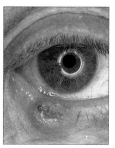

Basal cell carcinoma
This is the most common skin cancer and usually occurs on the face. It often has rolled edges and a central depression, which may become ulcerated.

General examination
Get to know what your skin looks like, using a mirror to examine areas you cannot see. Note the location of your most prominent moles and count them. You might consider making a mole "map" (below), marking the location of selected moles on a drawing or photograph of yourself.

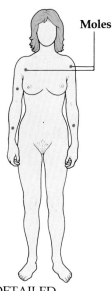

Moles

DETAILED EXAMINATION

1 Make a systematic examination of the upper part of your body, working up your arms to your shoulders. Look at all areas carefully and feel for any roughening. Examine any suspicious moles through a magnifying glass.

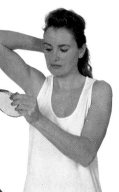

2 Closely examine your face and neck, running your fingers over your face to feel for rough areas. Most skin cancers start in this area, so be thorough. If you are a man, make sure you check under facial hair.

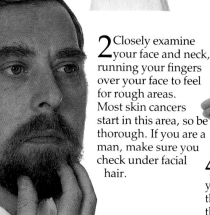

3 Use two mirrors to examine your scalp, the back of your neck, and your shoulders. Then move down the entire length of your back, across your buttocks, and down your legs. Your partner or a friend could help with this part of the examination.

4 Examine the front of your legs and your feet, including the soles and between the toes. Look for dark spots under your fingernails and toenails. Dark spots can be a sign of malignant melanoma.

Severe, persistent headaches

Headaches can have many causes. They are rarely due to a serious disease but are often related to stress, causing the well-known tension headache. In older people, headaches can indicate temporal arteritis, inflammation of the walls of the arteries that pass over the temples in the scalp. But headaches can also indicate a benign or malignant brain tumor, especially if they occur in a child and are progressively more severe or accompanied by any neurological symptoms such as lack of coordination, muscle weakness, or disturbance of vision or hearing.

Unusual bumps or lumps

See the symptoms chart on page 68.

Swallowing difficulties

Many ailments, including the common cold, swollen glands, or tonsillitis, can cause difficulty swallowing. Cancer of the esophagus may be the cause of this symptom if the swallowing difficulty is persistent and gets worse, so that it gradually causes you to have difficulty swallowing solids, then soft foods, and finally liquids.

Persistent hoarseness

See the symptoms chart on page 73.

Coughing up blood

Coughing up blood-stained phlegm can be caused by several conditions, including bronchitis or another chest infection. However, if the cough persists for many weeks or months, it could be due to lung cancer, especially in a person who smokes or once smoked. Never ignore a cough accompanied by blood; call your doctor immediately.

Persistent abdominal pain

Most pain in the abdomen is caused by minor digestive problems. However, if the pain is recurrent, lasts more than 48 hours, or is accompanied by other symptoms, seek medical attention. The cause could be a disorder such as irritable bowel syndrome, an ulcer, or inflammation that involves other abdominal organs such as the gallbladder, appendix, ovaries, or bladder. However, less frequently, the pain may be caused by a cancer in the abdomen.

Blood in the urine

Natural or artificial food colorings can sometimes pass into the urine, giving the appearance of blood. For example, after eating beets some people pass red urine. Urine that is pink, red, or smoke-colored could indicate the presence of blood (hematuria). This may be a sign of cancer

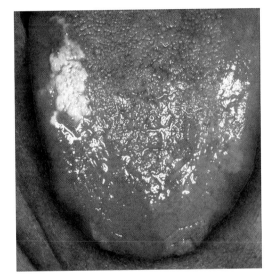

Leukoplakia
A whitish patch, known as leukoplakia, that appears anywhere in your mouth should be reported to your doctor. Although not actually cancerous, if left untreated it may develop into cancer. Leukoplakia usually results from chronic irritation due to smoking, poor dental hygiene, or badly fitting dentures.

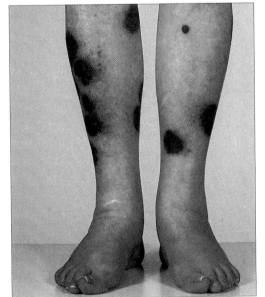

Purpura
Unexplained bruising of the skin (purpura) can have many causes but is sometimes a sign of leukemia; purpura should be brought to the attention of your doctor.

of the bladder or kidney, especially if there is no pain. Hematuria that is accompanied by pain is more likely to be a sign of infection or inflammation of the urinary tract, or of a kidney or bladder stone. However, all instances in which blood in the urine occurs should be brought to the attention of your doctor as soon as possible.

Change in bowel habits

An abrupt change in your bowel habits that cannot be explained by a minor illness or a change in your diet should always be investigated; it may indicate a cancer of the intestines. Benign conditions that can cause such changes include irritable bowel syndrome, hemorrhoids, anal fissures (tears in the lining of the anal canal), diverticular disease, or inflammation such as Crohn's disease or ulcerative colitis.

Rectal bleeding

The most common cause of rectal bleeding is hemorrhoids, which are swollen veins in the lining of the anus. If the blood is bright red and noticeable on the toilet paper or on the surface of the feces, or drips into the toilet bowl, you may have hemorrhoids. However, if blood is mixed in with the feces or if you have a change in your bowel habits, cancer is a possibility. In any instance of rectal bleeding, see your doctor.

Nonmenstrual bleeding

Vaginal bleeding between periods or after the menopause may be due to cancer of the cervix or uterus. However, it is also a sign of cervical erosion, a condition in which the surface lining of the cervix is more fragile than normal and tends to bleed. Vaginal bleeding can also be caused by an infection of the cervix or by cervical polyps. Women who take oral contraceptives sometimes experience "spotting" between periods, which may indicate that a change to a different type of oral contraceptive is advisable. If you experience any vaginal bleeding, report it to your doctor.

TESTICLE SELF-EXAMINATION

Cancer of the testicle is the most common cancer in men in the 20- to 35-year age group. Those particularly at risk are young white males who have a history of an undescended testicle. If detected early, testicular cancer is one of the most easily curable of all cancers. Self-examination should be performed monthly or more often. Feel for any enlargement or irregularity of your testicles. Perform the examination after a bath or shower when the scrotal skin is relaxed.

What to feel for
A cancerous tumor usually begins as a small, painless, hard, pealike bump like a pebble embedded in the surface of the testicle. A soft, painless swelling is more likely to be a harmless cyst. Painful swellings may be due to infection of the testicle or epididymis. Don't take any chances. See your doctor immediately if you detect any changes in your testicles.

How to examine your testicles
Examine each testicle separately, holding it in both hands and gently feeling all areas by rolling it between your fingers and thumb. Spend about 30 seconds to 1 minute per testicle.

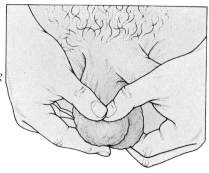

Testicle

Tumor

Epididymis

Scrotum

MONITOR YOUR SYMPTOMS
PERSISTENT HOARSENESS

Hoarseness or loss of voice is most often a result of laryngitis (inflammation of the voice box). This may be due to many common infections, such as the common cold or flu, or to overuse of the voice, and usually responds to resting the voice. However, if hoarseness lasts longer than a week or is recurrent, it may indicate a more serious underlying disorder, including several types of cancer. Always seek your doctor's advice in such cases.

HOARSENESS IN CHILDREN

A child who is hoarse and has a "barking" cough and wheezing may be suffering from croup (inflammation and narrowing of the air passages). The condition is very common in children up to 4 years. It is usually mild and of short duration but could be serious if accompanied by a high fever.

BEGIN HERE

Are you a heavy drinker and smoker?

YES ▷ **Heavy drinking and smoking** may cause chronic irritation of the larynx, leading to persistent hoarseness, loss of voice, and possibly cancer.

Action Consult your doctor. If irritation of the larynx is confirmed, you will be advised to stop smoking and drinking. You will need to eliminate these habits if you are to avoid permanent damage or cancer.

Severe hoarseness or loss of voice in the absence of other symptoms usually indicates a problem with the larynx.
Have you been using your voice a lot?

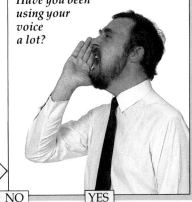

NO

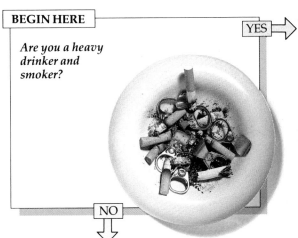

An underactive thyroid gland (hypothyroidism) is uncommon but can be a cause of persistent hoarseness, particularly in middle-aged women.
Are you over 40 and have you had two or more of the following symptoms?
◆ *Increased sensitivity to cold*
◆ *Dry skin or hair*
◆ *Weight gain without increased food intake*

NO ▷ **The abrupt onset of persistent hoarseness or loss of voice possibly combined with a chronic cough always needs investigation.**
Have you been hoarse for more than 3 weeks and do you have other chest symptoms such as coughing, wheezing, or shortness of breath?

NO ▷

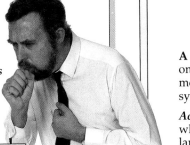

NO

YES

A polyp (a benign growth) on your vocal cords is the most likely cause of your symptoms.

Action Consult your doctor, who will examine your larynx to rule out cancer.

YES

Hypothyroidism could be the problem.

Action Consult your doctor. If hypothyroidism is suspected, tests will be performed to confirm the diagnosis.

YES

CONSULT YOUR DOCTOR WITHOUT DELAY!

You may have a lung infection but lung cancer is also possible.

Action After a thorough physical examination, samples of blood and phlegm will probably be taken for analysis. You may also have a chest X-ray. If cancer is suspected, other tests may also be performed.

CONSULT YOUR DOCTOR WITHOUT DELAY!

Cancer of the larynx could be causing your hoarseness regardless of the way you use your voice.

Action The doctor will examine your throat and a sample of tissue may be taken for examination under a microscope.

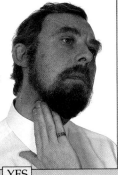

BREAST SELF-EXAMINATION

The American Cancer Society recommends that all women over the age of 20 perform monthly breast self-examinations. The best time is at the end of the menstrual period when the breasts are not swollen or tender. After the menopause, any easy-to-remember date will do, such as the first of each month. Use the same technique each time you examine your breasts, and examine both breasts in the same way so that any changes will be immediately obvious. If you find a lump, consult your doctor immediately. About four out of five breast lumps are found to be benign.

VISUAL INSPECTION

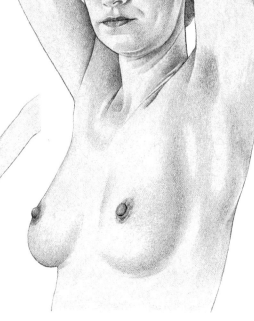

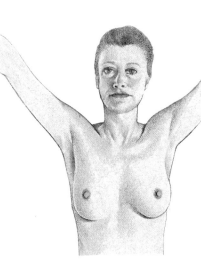

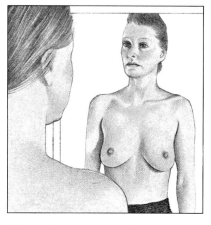

1 Begin by standing in front of a mirror with your arms at your sides. You should be checking for any changes, such as those shown in the box at lower right.

2 Lift your arms and turn from side to side, so that you can see all of each breast. Look carefully for dimples and other changes.

3 Place your hands behind your head to stretch the skin of your breasts, and again turn from side to side looking for changes. Inspect the undersides especially carefully.

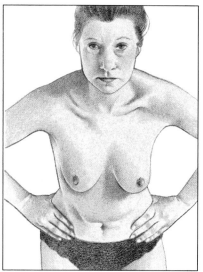

WHAT TO LOOK FOR

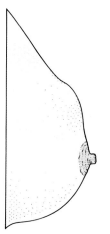

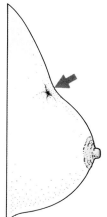

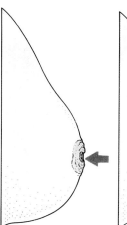

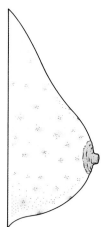

4 Finally, lean forward with your hands pressing down on your hips to flex your chest muscles and inspect the top surfaces of your breasts.

Change in breast contour, such as a swelling

Change in direction of the nipple

Dimpling or puckering of the skin

"Orange-peel" appearance of breast skin

FEELING FOR LUMPS

Lie on your back with a pillow or folded towel under one shoulder and the arm on that side placed behind your head. Using the pads of the middle three fingers of the other hand, start feeling your breasts just above the nipple on the outer part of the breast, and move around the breast, feeling every part, using one of the techniques shown below. Repeat the same procedure on the other breast. You should spend a minimum of 2 minutes on each breast, more if you have large breasts.

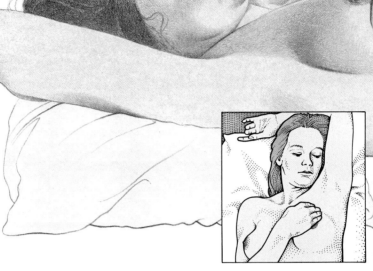

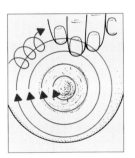

Technique
Press down gently, using small dime-sized circular motions to feel for any thickening of tissue or for lumps. Gradually move your hand in a series of circles around the breast, until you have felt the entire breast.

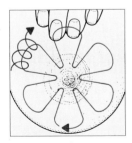

For large breasts
Make small circular movements from the 12 o'clock position down toward the nipple, and out toward the 1 o'clock position. Repeat for all "clock hand" positions.

Feeling for armpit lumps
After you have worked around the entire breast, feel the armpit for any lumps or swellings.

CHECKING FOR NIPPLE DISCHARGE

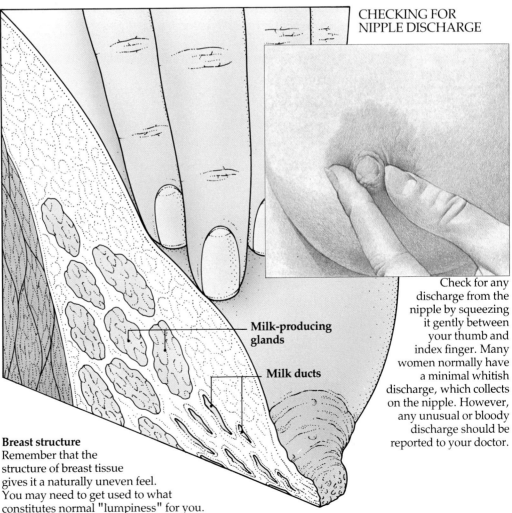

Milk-producing glands

Milk ducts

Breast structure
Remember that the structure of breast tissue gives it a naturally uneven feel. You may need to get used to what constitutes normal "lumpiness" for you.

Check for any discharge from the nipple by squeezing it gently between your thumb and index finger. Many women normally have a minimal whitish discharge, which collects on the nipple. However, any unusual or bloody discharge should be reported to your doctor.

CANCER SCREENING

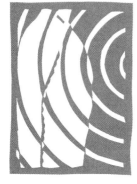

IN ADDITION TO REGULAR self-examinations and increased personal awareness of potentially cancerous changes, professional cancer screening provides another important means of detecting cancer at an early stage. Cancer screening involves testing groups of apparently healthy people with the goal of detecting cancer at an early stage, when treatment is likely to be most effective.

Experts in cancer research report that cancer screening must fulfill certain conditions to be worthwhile. It must be easy to administer, acceptable to the patient, cause a minimum of discomfort, and be priced within reason. Also essential is a reasonable level of accuracy. Finally, the facilities needed to conduct a full follow-up investigation and any necessary treatment must be readily available and it must be known that early treatment improves the chances of a complete cure.

TYPES OF SCREENING TESTS

The cancers that have lent themselves most successfully to screening on a large scale are those of the breast and the cervix (the neck of the uterus), mainly because the breast and cervix can be repeatedly examined safely and easily and because these cancers often progress in a deliberate fashion, thus facilitating detection at an early stage. Screening for

CERVICAL (PAP) SMEAR TEST

This test is used in the prevention and early detection of cancer of the cervix (the neck of the uterus). It involves taking cells from the cervix and examining them under a microscope to detect any abnormal changes. The procedure is risk-free, painless, quick, and 95 percent accurate in detecting dysplasia (the presence of abnormal cells), which, if not detected and treated, could develop into cancer.

HOW IT IS DONE

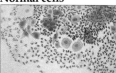

Normal cells

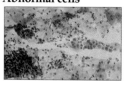

Abnormal cells

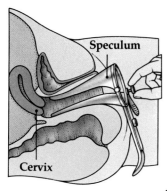

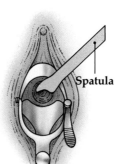

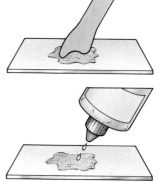

1 The woman lies on her back with her knees bent. She is asked to relax and let her knees fall open. A speculum is inserted into the vagina to hold it open.

2 A spatula and a cotton swab are inserted through the vagina to scrape some cells from the surface of the cervix.

3 The cells obtained from the cervix are smeared on a glass slide, fixed, and stained with dye.

4 The prepared cells are examined under a microscope and graded as normal, abnormal, or cancerous. Treatment is planned accordingly.

lung cancer has been less successful. There are also early detection tests for colon and rectal cancers, which are recommended much more frequently for those who are at high risk. There are myriad other screening tests, but many are suitable only for selective follow-up of high-risk groups, such as chest X-rays for people who have been exposed to asbestos.

Cancer of the cervix

The cervical (Pap) smear test is perhaps the most striking example of successful screening. Its widespread introduction halved the incidence of cervical cancer in the US from 1945 to 1975 (though there is some evidence that the incidence was beginning to decline before the introduction of the cervical smear). The test is now universally recommended as a means of detecting both the precancerous stage and a very early cancer of the cervix. Little official agreement has been reached on how often cervical smears should be done. Recommendations vary. The Canadian Task Force recommends that an examination be done every 3 years up to age 35, then once every 5 years thereafter. The American College of Obstetrics and Gynecology and the American Cancer Society recommend that an examination be done once a year

SCREENING TESTS FOR CANCER

This table presents the guidelines of the American Cancer Society for professional screening tests. The recommendations are for symptom-free people; they do not address factors that might indicate an increased risk. Ask your doctor if you think you could be in a higher risk category.

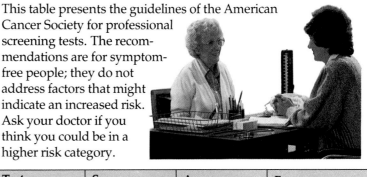

Test or procedure	Sex	Age	Frequency
Cervical (Pap) smear	Women	All women 18 or older; all women who are sexually active	Every year; every 3 years after three negative examinations
Mammography	Women	Between 35 and 39 40 to 49 Over 50	Once Every 1 to 2 years Every year
Digital rectal examination	Men and women	Over 40	Every year
Fecal occult blood test	Men and women	Over 50	Every year
Sigmoidoscopy	Men and women	Over 50	Every 3 to 5 years after two negative examinations done 1 year apart

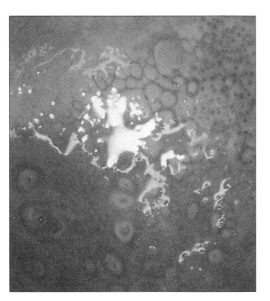

Colposcopy
If a cervical (Pap) smear shows abnormal cells, the cervix is examined directly by colposcopy, in which a speculum is inserted into the vagina to expose the cervix so that it can be examined under magnification. A solution applied to the cervix highlights any abnormal areas (as shown at left). A biopsy of the areas can be taken to determine whether the cells are precancerous or cancerous.

for all women over the age of 18. Your doctor can recommend how often you should have an examination.

Multiple sex partners and an early age of first sexual intercourse are risk factors for cervical cancer, making regular cervical smears especially important. Women whose mothers took diethylstilbestrol (DES) are also at high risk (see page 60).

Breast cancer

The results of screening for breast cancer have been encouraging. In one study, 20,000 women aged 40 to 64 were examined by doctors and by mammography (X-ray). The mortality from breast cancer

CASE HISTORY
A SMALL LUMP IN THE BREAST

WHILE SHOWERING, JOAN **felt a small, firm lump in the upper outer portion of her right breast. She had been examining her breasts at the same time every month for several years and was familiar with the shape and feel of her breasts. She had never felt this lump before, however. She went to see her doctor immediately.**

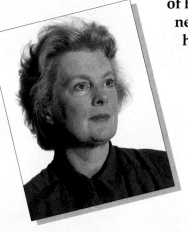

PERSONAL DETAILS
Name Joan Schering
Age 51
Occupation Professional musician
Family Joan's mother died of breast cancer at the age of 61.

MEDICAL BACKGROUND
Joan has been treated over a period of years for dyspepsia and peptic ulceration. Her condition had improved recently after taking a new antiulcer drug.

THE CONSULTATION
The doctor examines both breasts. There is no puckering of the skin, but he is able to feel the mass. He is pleased to note that the lump moves freely and does not seem to adhere to the underlying chest wall. He carefully feels both armpits and is relieved to find no swelling of the lymph glands.

The doctor tells Joan that she must have a mammogram and schedules it for the same day. The test confirms that there is a small, well-localized mass. The doctor recommends an immediate biopsy, which is performed in the outpatient department of the hospital.

THE DIAGNOSIS
The surgeon tells Joan that the biopsy has confirmed BREAST CANCER. He explains that additional tests will help determine whether any spread has occurred. Joan has several blood tests and other studies, including a bone and a liver scan; the results are negative. The surgeon tells her that he would like to perform an operation as soon as possible.

He says that, since the lump is so small, he recommends removing only the lump (lumpectomy) and the glands in her armpit. This will be followed by radiation therapy to her breast and armpit.

THE TREATMENT
Joan is admitted to the hospital. The lump is removed through a small incision that leaves a slight depression in her breast. The pathology report on the removed tumor suggests that the surgeon has removed all of the tumor. Three days later she attends her first radiation therapy session. She has radiation therapy five times a week for a month. The skin of her breast becomes slightly reddened and later looks tanned and slightly thickened.

THE OUTCOME
Joan completes her radiation therapy and is able to return to orchestral playing 3 to 4 weeks later. She remains well and, although at first apprehensive about the prospect of a recurrence, is apparently free of cancer and leading an active life 5 years later. Joan is convinced that she owes her life to the early detection and treatment of her cancer. She continues her monthly self-examinations.

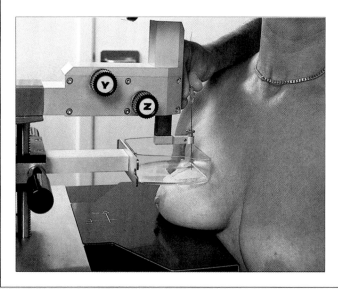

Diagnosis and treatment
Joan's diagnosis is confirmed by a needle biopsy, in which a small piece of tissue is removed by inserting a needle through the skin (left). Treatment of Joan's tumor is by lumpectomy, in which the lump and a small margin of surrounding skin are removed.

PROCEDURE FOR MAMMOGRAPHY

Mammography, or breast X-ray, can detect breast cancer before any lumps can be felt. In the procedure shown here, one breast at a time is positioned on an X-ray film and a plastic cover is used to flatten the breast gently against the plate. Two or three different views are usually taken.

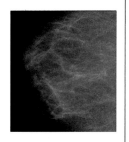

Normal breast
This mammogram shows a healthy breast. The denser, white areas are milk ducts.

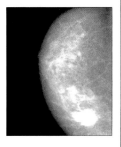

Breast tumor
The dense white area at the bottom of this mammogram indicates a tumor. A biopsy is needed to determine whether it is cancerous.

among the screened women 10 years after they started the study was reduced by about 25 percent in comparison to an equivalent group of women who were not screened; there had been 146 deaths from breast cancer in the screened group and 192 deaths from the same cause in the unscreened group. About one third of the breast cancers detected by mammography were in the early stage.

There is very little controversy about the value of mammography; equipment and techniques have improved in recent years as experience in the interpretation of the images has grown. However, mammography cannot definitively diagnose cancer. Mammography highlights those areas, often before a lump can be felt, in which cancer might be present and which require further investigation (such as a biopsy).

Colon and rectal cancer

The simplest screening test for cancer of the rectum is the digital rectal examination (see right). The American Cancer Society recommends that the test be done yearly for men and women over 40. This examination may also detect cancer of the prostate at an early stage.

Cancers of the colon and rectum frequently produce very slight bleeding. This blood loss is not great enough to be seen in the stools, but is enough to be detected by a sensitive test using paper

Digital rectal examination
The patient usually lies on his or her left side with knees bent toward the chest. The doctor inserts a gloved, lubricated finger into the rectum to feel for any abnormalities. In men, because the prostate can be felt through the rectum, it is also possible to check for cancer of the prostate. Examination of the prostate may also be performed with the patient standing and bent at the waist, as shown at left.

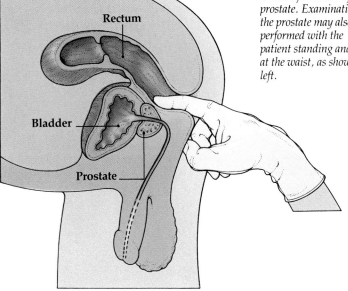

Rectum

Bladder

Prostate

ASK YOUR DOCTOR
CANCER SCREENING

Q A friend of mine had a mammogram that showed no signs of cancer. However, 2 years later, she was diagnosed as having breast cancer. Is mammography really reliable?

A Mammography cannot predict the development of cancer, but it can reliably detect a growth in the breast once it has reached a certain size, and often before it can be felt. A rapidly growing tumor may become apparent between mammograms. The discovery of tumors depends in part on the frequency of examinations.

Q My husband is going to have some tests done and I am wondering what will happen if the test results are positive. Will he get treatment right away?

A Tests are the first stage in diagnosis. A positive result will lead to a biopsy and possibly more tests to evaluate your husband's condition.

Q There is a history of cancer of the colon in my family. Does this mean that I need to have extra screening tests?

A Anyone who has a parent or sibling in whom cancer of the colon or rectum developed before the age of 50 is at increased risk of colorectal cancer. So are those with ulcerative colitis or a family background of polyps in the colon. All these people should have more frequent screening examinations, starting at an earlier age than the general population. Your doctor will advise you when to start having tests.

Fecal occult blood test
A small sample of stool is placed on a piece of filter paper. Chemicals are then added to the mixture; if the mixture turns blue, there may be blood in the stool.

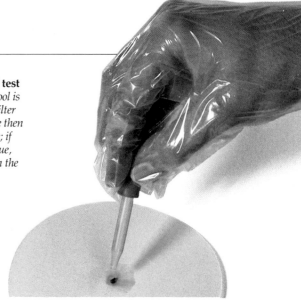

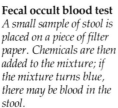

impregnated with a chemical indicator. Known as the fecal occult blood test, this screening tool is simple to perform, accurate in the hands of a doctor or a trained technician, inexpensive, and quick. It is recommended that men and women over 50 have the test annually.

Some authorities maintain that screening for blood in the stools is not enough. Since the majority (more than 90 percent) of cancers of the colon or rectum originate in polyps in the bowels of people over 50, it seems to make sense to look for polyps. This can be done by using a fiberoptic endoscope, a flexible tube with a light on the end. Because the examination extends up through and occasionally just beyond the sigmoid colon, it is called sigmoidoscopy. If everyone over 50 were examined periodically with these three procedures, it is possible that the majority of colon and rectal cancers could be detected at an early and curable stage and that some could be avoided altogether.

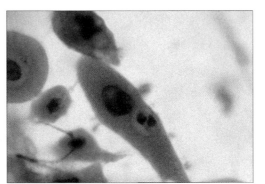

Sputum
This microscope view of a sputum sample reveals a malignant cell (orange) that has been shed from a tumor in the lung. However, sputum tests do not usually detect lung cancer at a treatable stage (before the tumor has spread).

CASE HISTORY
BLOOD IN THE STOOLS

T ONY HAD NOTICED BRIGHT RED BLOOD **on the surface of his stools. Concerned, he made an appointment to see his doctor the next day. There was no pain during his bowel movements and Tony had not noticed any other change in the appearance of his stools. He hoped that the cause of the bleeding was nothing more serious than hemorrhoids. Nevertheless, because there was a history of cancer in his family, Tony felt anxious about what the doctor might find.**

PERSONAL DETAILS
Name Tony Williams
Age 61
Occupation Restaurateur
Family One of Tony's brothers died of cancer of the colon.

MEDICAL BACKGROUND
Tony's health is generally good. His only major problem has been intermittent attacks of pain in the lower part of his back attributed to degenerative joint disease.

THE CONSULTATION
Tony tells the doctor about his symptoms and asks whether the cause could be hemorrhoids. The doctor says that it is possible but, taking into account Tony's age and family history, he wants to perform a rectal examination. The doctor performs the examination and feels something firm in the uppermost part of the rectum. Tony's doctor refers him to a gastroenterologist – a doctor who performs examinations of the colon and rectum by fiberoptic sigmoidoscopy and colonoscopy.

FURTHER INVESTIGATION
The colonoscopic examination is performed under mild sedation and causes Tony very little discomfort. One large polyp, almost 1.5 inches in diameter, and numerous small ones are found in the upper part of the rectum. The large polyp is ulcerated and is the cause of the bleeding. No other polyps are found in the rest of the colon.

THE DIAGNOSIS
Biopsy confirms the diagnosis of a RECTAL CANCER situated high up in the rectum. The pathologist reports that appearances suggest that the tumor cells are confined to the head of the large polyp and may not have spread widely. The doctor tells Tony that the cancer has been detected at a relatively early stage. He says that, since 90 percent of colorectal cancers arise from polyps, everyone over 50 is advised to have screening for polyps; those with a family history of colorectal cancer should have screenings from the age of 40.

THE TREATMENT
Tony needs surgery to eliminate all traces of cancer. Only a short segment of his bowel is removed and the ends are joined by stapling, so Tony does not need to have a colostomy. He is able to return to work within 2 months of his operation and, if he sees his doctor regularly, has at least a 90 percent chance of avoiding a recurrence.

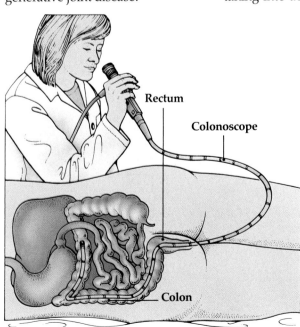

Colonoscopic examination
A flexible tube with a light on the end – a colonoscope – is used to examine the internal lining of Tony's rectum and colon. The photograph below, taken through the instrument, shows several polyps found in the rectum.

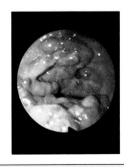

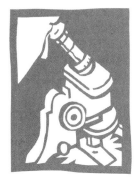

DIAGNOSIS AND ASSESSMENT

U LTIMATELY, ALL CANCER DIAGNOSES rely on examination of a specimen of the abnormal tissue – a biopsy – in the laboratory by a pathologist. However, a doctor may also use other tests to establish the presence of a malignant tumor or to assess the extent of its spread. Both considerations have significant implications for the patient who will undergo treatment.

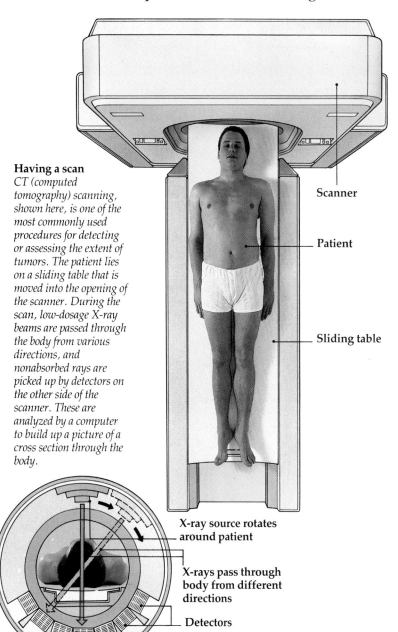

Having a scan
CT (computed tomography) scanning, shown here, is one of the most commonly used procedures for detecting or assessing the extent of tumors. The patient lies on a sliding table that is moved into the opening of the scanner. During the scan, low-dosage X-ray beams are passed through the body from various directions, and nonabsorbed rays are picked up by detectors on the other side of the scanner. These are analyzed by a computer to build up a picture of a cross section through the body.

Scanner

Patient

Sliding table

X-ray source rotates around patient

X-rays pass through body from different directions

Detectors

A diagnosis of cancer may be reached by several routes. At first, there is usually only a suspicion of cancer. The suspicion may have been aroused by one or more physical signs or symptoms that have prompted a person to visit the doctor. For example, there may be a lump, unexplained bleeding, or an unexplainable loss of weight. In other cases, a screening test, such as mammography, may have aroused the doctor's suspicions.

IMAGING

If the patient has an obvious lump, the diagnostic process often moves directly to taking a biopsy of the suspicious area or to removal of the lump in its entirety.

In other cases, different tests may be needed to determine the cause of symptoms and signs. Often, a part of the body requires imaging (see IMAGING TUMORS on pages 84 and 85). Sometimes a flexible viewing instrument, an endoscope, is used to look inside the body (see ENDOSCOPY at right). When a tumor is within range of direct endoscopic inspection and biopsy, it may allow the diagnosis to be confirmed.

BIOPSIES

The final diagnosis of cancer can be made only by taking a piece of the abnormal tissue from the body (a biopsy) and by examining it under a microscope.

ENDOSCOPY

Endoscopy is the use of a viewing instrument to look inside the body. Endoscopes, which may be flexible or rigid, include gastroscopes, colonoscopes, and sigmoidoscopes for examining the digestive tract; bronchoscopes to look at the large airways in the lungs; cystoscopes for examining the inside of the bladder; and laparoscopes for examining the lower part of the abdomen.

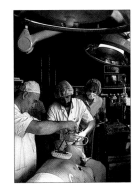

Bronchoscopy
During bronchoscopy, a flexible endoscope is passed beyond the larynx into the windpipe and into the large airways in the lungs. This type of examination is used for the detection of lung cancer.

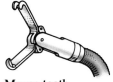

Mouse-tooth forceps

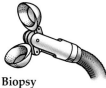

Biopsy forceps

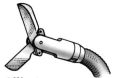

Alligator forceps

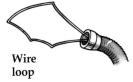

Wire loop

Attachment to light source

Eyepiece

Cable tip control

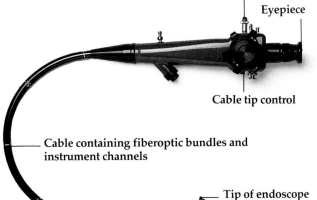

Cable containing fiberoptic bundles and instrument channels

Tip of endoscope

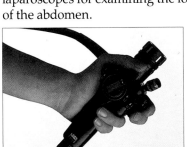

Parts of a flexible endoscope
A flexible endoscope consists of a light source, an eyepiece, and a flexible cable. Light rays pass along fiberoptic bundles in the cable, illuminate the area, and pass back up the cable to the viewer. The endoscope also contains channels through which instruments (right) can be passed to take tissue samples.

BIOPSIES

Biopsy is the removal of a sample of tissue from the body for examination under a microscope. Biopsies are performed to distinguish nonmalignant tumors from malignant ones. A biopsy can be performed in a variety of ways; the method selected depends on where the tumor is and the amount of tissue needed to make a diagnosis.

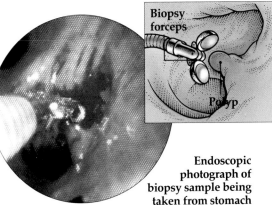

Biopsy forceps

Polyp

Endoscopic photograph of biopsy sample being taken from stomach

1 An endoscopic biopsy (shown here) is taken via an endoscope. For an excisional biopsy, a lump is removed using a scalpel or other cutting device. For a needle biopsy, a thin hollow needle is inserted into the body and some cells are sucked out or a thin core of tissue is taken.

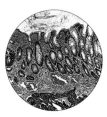

Cancer cells
This photograph of a biopsy specimen shows cancer of the stomach.

2 Solid tissue samples are embedded in wax, giving them a firm consistency suitable for slicing. This process usually takes several days. The sample may be frozen before slicing if a diagnosis is urgently needed.

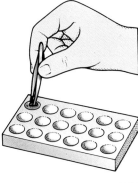

3 The tissue sample is cut into ultrathin slices and mounted on a microscope slide. Nonsolid tissue samples (usually obtained by needle biopsy) are smeared directly onto a microscope slide and then fixed and stained for viewing.

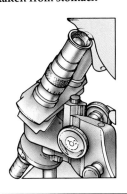

IMAGING TUMORS

Many types of imaging procedures may be used to detect primary tumors or to look for any spread of a cancer to sites beyond the original tumor (secondary sites). Images produced by seven different techniques are shown here. All the techniques are safe (except for the very small risks – justified by the danger of missing a cancer – from X-ray procedures) and involve minimal or no discomfort. For a **plain X-ray**, the part of the body to be imaged is placed between an X-ray source and a radiosensitive film. When the film is developed, some solid tumors appear as lighter areas within darker normal tissue. In **contrast X-ray imaging**, a contrast medium that absorbs X-rays is introduced into the body. This medium helps doctors see tumors in organs such as the colon. **CT scanning** uses X-rays that are passed through the body from many directions and analyzed

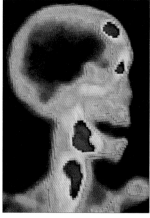

Bone cancer
The color-enhanced radionuclide scan above shows several tumors in the bones of the head and neck (red areas). These are secondary tumors, caused by spread of cancer cells from another part of the body.

Eye muscle cancer
The image at right, obtained by CT scanning, shows a tumor (a rhabdomyosarcoma) of a muscle of the right eye (arrow). The tumor has spread around the surface of the eye.

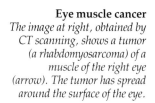

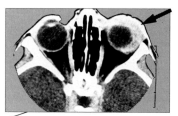

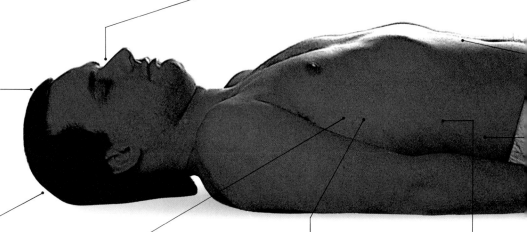

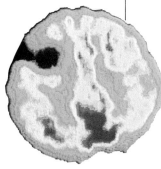

Brain tumor
The image above is a color-enhanced PET scan showing a cross section through the brain. The tumor is represented by the black area at top left.

Hodgkin's disease
The color-enhanced image below, obtained by MRI, shows a chest cross section. The white areas represent fluid collection around the lungs and heart, a feature of advanced Hodgkin's disease.

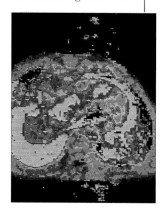

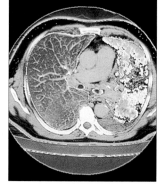

Lung cancer
The image above shows a cross section through the chest obtained by CT scanning. The scan reveals a dramatic difference between the healthy right lung (left on image) and the cancerous left lung.

Liver cancer
The radionuclide scan below shows the liver as the dark area on the left. The patchy pale areas in the liver correspond to secondary tumors.

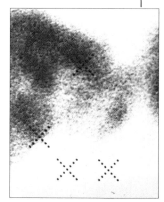

by a computer to produce a cross-sectional image.

Other scanning techniques also use computer technology. In **radionuclide scanning**, radioisotopes are introduced into the body and the radiation they emit is detected. This technique may reveal tumors that absorb more or less of the radioisotope than normal tissues. **Positron emission tomography (PET) scanning** is a type of radionuclide scan that uses special isotopes to produce a cross-sectional image. The image shows the structure or even the function of certain tissues. **Ultrasound scanning** works by passing high-frequency sound waves into the body and detecting their echoes from body structures. In **magnetic resonance imaging (MRI)**, imaging is based on the detection of radio signals from atoms in the body when the body is placed in a strong magnetic field and bombarded with radio waves.

Osteosarcoma
The X-ray at right shows a type of bone cancer (an osteosarcoma) affecting the thighbone. The knee joint is below the bottom of the image. The tumor is represented by the fuzzy area around the solid white bone.

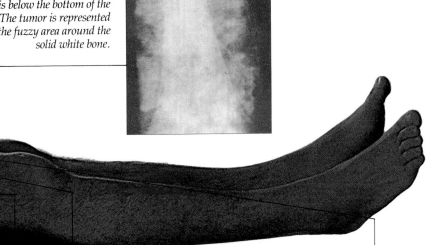

Bone cancer
The color-enhanced radionuclide scan of the pelvis, below, reveals a tumor (white area) in the head of the femur (thighbone), which forms part of the ball-and-socket hip joint.

Kidney tumor
The image below is an ultrasound scan of the abdomen. The rounded white area is a tumor in a kidney. The surrounding dark areas are normal kidney and liver tissue.

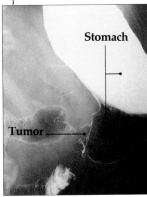

Stomach

Tumor

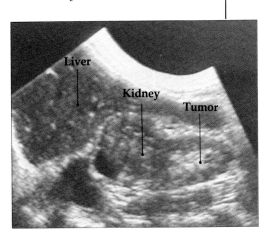

Liver

Kidney

Tumor

Stomach cancer
In the X-ray image above, the large white area is barium contrast medium filling the upper part of the stomach. The stomach is distended because a large tumor has obstructed the flow of the stomach contents into the intestines.

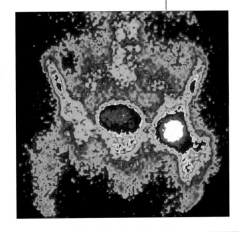

Excisional biopsy

This is the removal of all of a lump by an operation, with examination of the specimen for evidence of disease. Complete removal of a breast lump, to examine it for signs of cancer, is an example of an excisional biopsy. If the tumor is easily accessible, an excisional biopsy can be done using a local anesthetic. Occasionally a general anesthetic is needed.

Endoscopic biopsy

If a tumor is detected by means of an endoscope, a piece of tissue can usually be removed from it via the endoscope. Biopsies from tumors of the bladder, digestive tract, and airways in the lungs are often taken in this way. These procedures are usually done on an outpatient basis, often with the use of sedation rather than a general anesthetic.

STAGING BREAST CANCER

Both the size of the tumor and any indications that it has spread from the original site are evaluated in staging breast cancer. Five main stages are recognized, from carcinoma in situ, the most favorable, to stage IV, the least favorable. The treatment is affected by the stage at diagnosis; the survival rate is also affected by the stage.

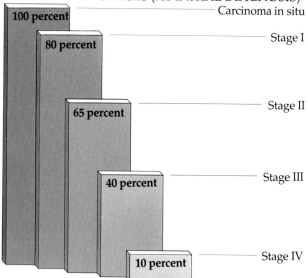

Stage I
Less than ¾ inch in diameter

Stage II
More than ¾ inch but less than 2 inches in diameter

Stage III
Larger than 2 inches in diameter

5-YEAR SURVIVAL RATES
OF DIFFERENT STAGES (AT INITIAL DIAGNOSIS)

- 100 percent — Carcinoma in situ
- 80 percent — Stage I
- 65 percent — Stage II
- 40 percent — Stage III
- 10 percent — Stage IV

Carcinoma in situ
In this stage, some normal cells have become malignant; however, they have not invaded adjacent cell groups. The 5-year survival rate is almost 100 percent.

Stage I
In this and subsequent stages, the tumor cells have grown into areas normally occupied by adjacent cells. The tumor is less than ¾ inch in diameter and the lymph glands under the arm are not affected. The survival rate 5 years after diagnosis is 80 percent.

Stage II
In stage II disease, the tumor is ¾ to 2 inches in diameter and lymph glands under the arm are either too small to feel or small and freely movable if felt. Patients are generally treated with surgery and chemotherapy.

Stage III
This stage is divided into Stage IIIA and IIIB. The tumor is larger than 2 inches and the cancer may have spread to the lymph glands under the arm and around the collarbone. Stage III disease is treated with combination therapy, often employing chemotherapy, surgery, and radiation therapy.

Stage IV
In stage IV disease, the tumor has spread beyond the breast and the local lymph glands to involve organs at sites around the body. Stage IV disease is treated with chemotherapy, although radiation therapy may also be used if the tumor involves the brain or causes painful bone lesions.

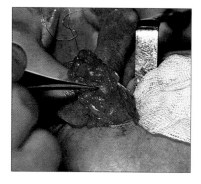

Lumpectomy
Breast cancers diagnosed at the stages of carcinoma-in-situ, Stage I, and Stage II can often be cured by lumpectomy. Apart from a small scar, there is no great change in the appearance of the affected breast.

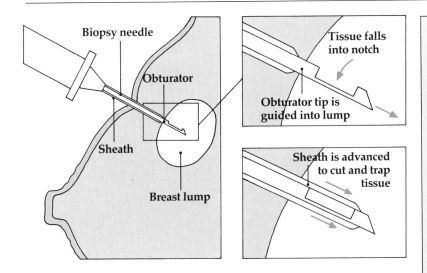

Biopsy needle

Obturator

Sheath

Breast lump

Tissue falls into notch

Obturator tip is guided into lump

Sheath is advanced to cut and trap tissue

STAGING

Once a diagnosis has been made, the doctor needs to know as much as possible about the tumor before recommending treatment. First, the doctor studies the patient's report and usually reviews the specimen with the pathologist who examined the abnormal tissue. The pathologist describes the nature of the cancer and its degree of malignancy. Because it is essential for the doctor to determine how far the cancer has spread, he or she may order more tests, including more imaging procedures and biopsies, if necessary.

The process of determining how advanced a cancer has become is called staging; staging has major implications for deciding on appropriate treatment. A cancer still confined to the site of origin can often be cured by surgical removal or radiation therapy. On the other hand, chemotherapy is the mainstay of therapy when a cancer has spread widely to other organs in the body. In the last instance, chemotherapy in association with surgery may be used. Through accurate staging, patients with widespread disease can be spared extensive surgery or radiation therapy that would not be useful.

An example of the staging of breast cancer is shown in the box at left.

Needle biopsy
To speed up and simplify the process of making a diagnosis, needle biopsy was developed. In this technique (shown above), a sample of tissue or some fluid and cells are obtained by means of a hollow needle inserted into the area of interest, such as a breast lump. Needle biopsy is quick, simple, and almost painless. Occasionally, an insufficient amount of material, or material of questionable diagnostic value, is obtained and an excisional biopsy is needed later.

ASK YOUR DOCTOR CANCER DIAGNOSIS

Q I have had two "positive" Pap tests. Does this mean I have cervical cancer? What happens next?

A Most probably, you do not have cancer. However, you may have precancerous changes in your cervix. The next step is to have a colposcopy (examination of the cervix with a special viewing instrument) and a biopsy. If these tests confirm precancerous changes (and if the biopsy itself has not removed the whole area of abnormality), your doctor will probably recommend minor surgery.

Q What is a bone marrow biopsy and how can it help in the diagnosis of cancer?

A Using a local anesthetic, a hollow needle is guided into the hipbone and a core of marrow is removed. The marrow is sometimes taken from the sternum (breastbone). The biopsy may reveal a cancer that affects the bone marrow (such as leukemia or multiple myeloma).

Q It was first suggested I might have cancer 3 weeks ago and the doctors are still running tests. Don't they realize how urgently I need treatment?

A Different cancers grow at strikingly different rates. Although it is important to act promptly, it is equally important to assess correctly the type and stage of cancer before beginning treatment. Your doctor will attempt to balance these sometimes conflicting goals as he or she completes the evaluation of your disease. If you have concerns about the time that the testing has required, talk with your doctor.

CHAPTER FIVE

CANCER TREATMENT

INTRODUCTION

SURGERY FOR CANCER

RADIATION THERAPY

CHEMOTHERAPY

UNCONVENTIONAL TREATMENT

T REATMENTS ARE AVAILABLE today for most forms of cancer and, fortunately, technology is advancing rapidly. In addition, success rates for these therapies are improving steadily. However, when cancer is diagnosed, treatment does not usually begin immediately. As quickly as possible, the oncologist (cancer specialist) or other doctor must gather all the relevant information. It may include the type and "aggressiveness" of the cancer, the extent of its spread, the patient's general health and ability to tolerate treatment, the side effects associated with available therapies, and the effectiveness of these therapies.

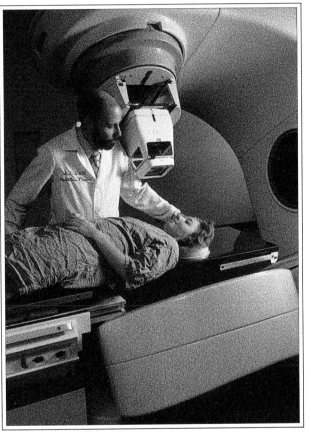

Once all the information has been collected, the doctor (or doctors) are in a position to decide which treatment options are available. It is crucial that the doctor and patient decide together what the goals of therapy are, taking into account the likelihood of success and the possibility of side effects. Sometimes these decisions are straightforward. For example, a woman who has a small, operable, breast cancer may choose between a mastectomy and a lumpectomy, followed by radiation therapy. Whatever the decision, the surgeon will examine the lymph glands under her arm for evidence of tumor spread. The oncologist may recommend a course of adjuvant chemotherapy – chemotherapy administered just after the tumor has been surgically removed. For most women, the chances of cure are good. With widely spread, aggressive cancers, the patient will have a choice among different strategies for palliative treatment (treatment that alleviates the symptoms, offering relief but not cure). Some of these strategies may be designed to extend survival; others simply improve the quality of life that remains.

The first two sections of this chapter, SURGERY FOR CANCER and RADIATION THERAPY, discuss two forms of treatment that are of greatest value in the treatment of cancers that have not spread far beyond their point of origin. The third section, CHEMOTHERAPY, reviews whole-body treatments that are of greater value in treating cancers that have already spread from their point of origin or have the potential to spread. In addition to the three major treatments – surgery, radiation therapy, and chemotherapy – other therapies have been claimed by unorthodox practitioners to be of benefit to cancer patients; these are evaluated in the final section, UNCONVENTIONAL TREATMENT.

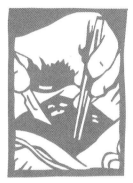

SURGERY FOR CANCER

S URGERY, RANGING FROM minor office procedures to major operations, may be required for cancer, depending on the type and severity of the disease. Overall, surgical treatments have cured more cancers than all other treatments combined. In addition, palliative operations are performed for some cancers even when a cure is not possible. Palliative surgery is performed to relieve or prevent the patient's distressing symptoms.

Surgeons are involved in at least part of the care of the majority of patients who have cancer. Even when chemotherapy (drug treatment) or radiation therapy is the mainstay of treatment, a minor operation (such as a biopsy) is often needed to obtain a sample of the cancerous tissue to make the diagnosis (see DIAGNOSIS AND ASSESSMENT on page 82).

SURGERY AIMED AT CURE

If a malignant tumor has remained truly localized, meaning that it has not spread to other parts of the body, surgical removal of the cancer can be curative. Because of this, surgery is usually the first option considered for many so-called solid

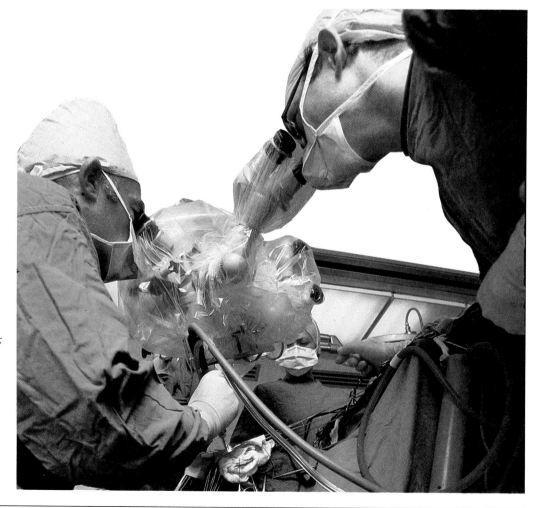

Removing a brain tumor
The surgeons in this photograph are using a special microscope that allows them to simultaneously view the operating area under magnification. The surgeon on the left is using an ultrasonic probe; ultrasonic vibrations emulsify (break up) the growth, allowing it to be sucked away. Tissue is removed from the center of the growth, causing it to collapse into itself, and allowing any remaining tumor matter to be more easily "teased" away from surrounding healthy tissue.

tumors (i.e., nearly all cancers except for leukemias and lymphomas), provided there are grounds for believing the cancer has not spread.

Before surgery

Surgery usually follows a biopsy, which is performed to confirm the diagnosis of cancer, and other noninvasive studies, which are performed to ascertain the stage of the cancer (how far it has spread). If the tumor is well localized, surgery is usually the first choice. The surgical options and implications of surgery are then reviewed by the surgeon with the patient and his or her family. This is the time to ask the surgeon any questions about preparation for surgery, the operation itself (its extent and effectiveness), and any risks and complications.

The days between the biopsy and the operation allow the patient a period of time for psychological adjustment and any physical preparation, such as treating other medical conditions.

Technique

Techniques used for removing tumors vary widely according to the site and extent of the tumor. Surgery today may be performed not with a scalpel but by electrosurgery – using an electrical current to cut through and/or remove tissue.

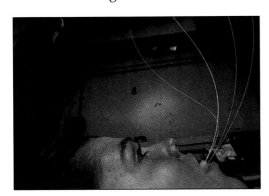

Laser treatment for throat cancer
In the photograph above, a red argon laser is being directed through four fiberoptic waveguides (conduits) to treat a malignant tumor in the patient's throat. The beams activate a drug, previously injected into the patient, that is highly toxic to cancerous cells.

UNDERSTANDING YOUR TREATMENT

Here is a checklist of questions to ask your surgeons if you have been advised to have surgery for cancer.

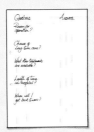

◆ Why is the operation being done and what will be removed?
◆ How will my body be affected after removal of this tissue or part of an organ?
◆ What is my chance of long-term cure?
◆ Are there alternative or less extensive treatments that might be available?
◆ How long will I be in the hospital?
◆ How long will it take before I get back to normal?
◆ How much pain and discomfort should I expect?
◆ What are the complications and risks of surgery?
◆ What help will I need when I get home?
◆ Will any other treatment be needed before or after surgical treatment?
◆ Is reconstructive surgery an option?
◆ What is the surgical team's experience with this procedure?

ASK YOUR DOCTOR
SURGERY FOR CANCER

Q Is it still common to diagnose cancer and remove the tumor during the same operation?

A Such one-step procedures are still sometimes performed because they spare the patient the risk of two anesthetics and of having more than one operation. However, it is now more common for a biopsy (removal of tissue from the tumor) to be performed first. The patient and doctors then discuss the results and possible treatments. Performing a biopsy before surgery gives the pathologist more time to provide a diagnosis. It also gives the patient time to adjust psychologically to the implications of surgery and more time to consider the treatment options.

Q My husband has prostate cancer, and his case will be presented to a tumor board. What is this?

A A tumor board is a group of cancer specialists, including surgical oncologists, radiation oncologists, and medical oncologists that meets to review and make recommendations regarding the management of individual cases of cancer.

Q Do doctors ever perform surgery to prevent cancer from developing?

A Yes. The most common example is treatment for a precancerous condition of the cervix. Another example concerns people with the inherited condition polyposis coli. A person affected by this disorder has hundreds of polyps in the colon. When the patient reaches his or her 30s, these polyps invariably turn malignant. The only way to prevent cancer is to remove the colon.

SURGICAL PROCEDURES
SURGERY FOR BREAST CANCER

FOUR DIFFERENT OPERATIONS for removal of a breast cancer are shown here, but there are several other variations. The operation recommended depends on the size and extent of the tumor, as well as on how it looks under a microscope. For tumors up to a certain stage, extensive surgery does not give a better chance of survival than a more conservative operation. Today, procedures such as lumpectomy, accompanied by radiation, are recommended more often. The patient and her surgeon should discuss breast reconstruction before a final decision about the choice of operation is made.

LUMPECTOMY

In this operation, only the tumor and a little surrounding tissue are removed. It is accompanied by removal of some lymph glands under the arm on the affected side. Lumpectomy is followed by radiation therapy and often by chemotherapy.

1 A small incision is made over the lump.

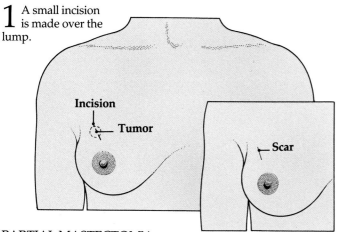

Incision — Tumor — Scar

2 The tumor and a small amount of the surrounding tissue are removed. The incision is closed.

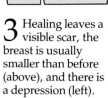

Tissue removed — Tumor — Small depression

3 Healing leaves a barely noticeable scar (left) and a small depression in the breast (above right).

PARTIAL MASTECTOMY

Here, a segment of breast tissue containing the tumor is removed. As with lumpectomy, some lymph glands in the armpit are also removed, and treatment with radiation therapy may follow.

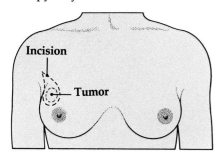

Incision — Tumor

2 The tumor and a segment of surrounding tissue and skin are removed. The incision is closed.

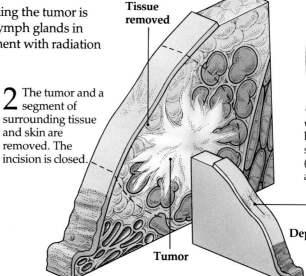

Tissue removed — Tumor

Scar

3 Healing leaves a visible scar, the breast is usually smaller than before (above), and there is a depression (left).

Depression

1 Incisions are made to cut out a segment of breast tissue and remove the lymph glands in the armpit as well.

SUBCUTANEOUS MASTECTOMY

In this operation, all of the inner tissue of the breast is removed, but the nipple and as much skin as possible are left. A silicone implant is then inserted. Lymph glands in the armpits are examined carefully, and some may be removed for biopsy. An alternative is for the skin and nipple to be removed as well (this is called a simple mastectomy). The breast is reconstructed later.

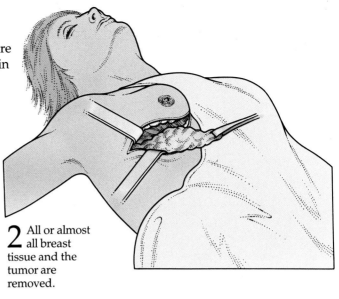

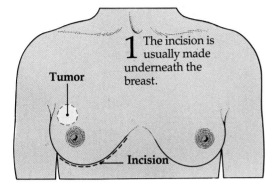

1 The incision is usually made underneath the breast.

Tumor

Incision

2 All or almost all breast tissue and the tumor are removed.

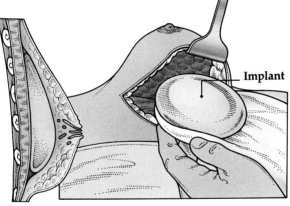

3 A silicone implant is inserted into the breast to restore appearance.

Implant

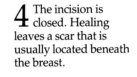

4 The incision is closed. Healing leaves a scar that is usually located beneath the breast.

MODIFIED RADICAL MASTECTOMY

The whole breast and all lymph glands under the arm are removed in a single block of tissue, if possible. The chest muscles are left in place. The breast can later be reconstructed. The chest muscles are rarely removed.

1 A large elliptical incision, encompassing the entire breast and extending into the armpit, is made. All breast tissue is cut out, down to the chest muscles, together with the lymph glands in the armpit. The incision is then closed.

Implant

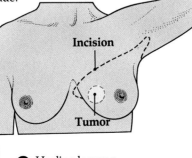

Incision

Tumor

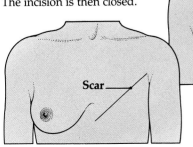

Scar

2 Healing leaves a long scar across the chest (left).

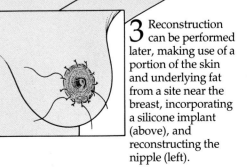

3 Reconstruction can be performed later, making use of a portion of the skin and underlying fat from a site near the breast, incorporating a silicone implant (above), and reconstructing the nipple (left).

SURGICAL PROCEDURES
REMOVAL OF A PROSTATE CANCER

S EVERAL DIFFERENT OPERATIONS **may be performed to treat prostate cancer. Some are augmented by radiation therapy. Of the operations shown below, the radical retropubic method can cure some prostate cancers. The transurethral method can relieve obstructive symptoms, but is not curative.**

TRANSURETHRAL PROSTATECTOMY

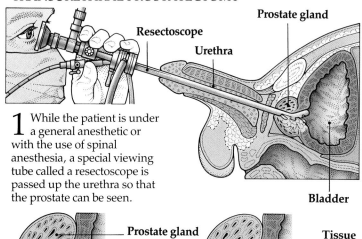

1 While the patient is under a general anesthetic or with the use of spinal anesthesia, a special viewing tube called a resectoscope is passed up the urethra so that the prostate can be seen.

2 A heated wire loop is inserted through the resectoscope and used to cut away at the tumor.

3 Sufficient tissue is cut away to relieve obstruction. The pieces of tissue are washed out through the resectoscope.

RADICAL RETROPUBIC PROSTATECTOMY

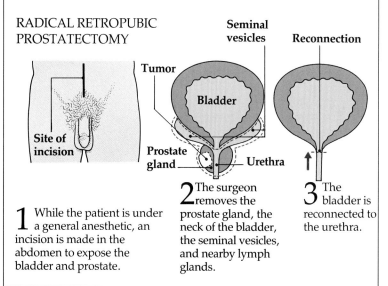

1 While the patient is under a general anesthetic, an incision is made in the abdomen to expose the bladder and prostate.

2 The surgeon removes the prostate gland, the neck of the bladder, the seminal vesicles, and nearby lymph glands.

3 The bladder is reconnected to the urethra.

Liquid nitrogen and other freezing techniques are often used to destroy cancers of the mouth, genitals, or skin. Laser surgery is used in the removal of some tumors of the rectum, female reproductive tract, and head and neck. Some bladder and prostate cancers are treated electrosurgically, by laser, or by another cutting tool inserted into the body via an endoscope (viewing instrument).

To offer the best chance of cure, the surgeon plans an operation that ensures that an adequate portion of healthy tissue is removed from the area around the tumor. The surgeon also removes any nearby lymph glands that may be affected. By removing these tissues, the surgeon can best achieve the removal of all the cancer. The amount of tissue cut out depends on the extent and location of the malignancy.

Outlook

A large percentage of operations performed to cure a cancer now achieve a cure. However, even sophisticated tests are not able to identify small collections of cancer cells in different parts of the body. If an operation is done after the cancer has already spread, these cells are likely to grow and the tumor will ultimately reappear at other sites such as the liver, lungs, or bone.

PALLIATIVE SURGERY

Palliative operations are designed to control the symptoms of cancer, rather than to cure it. For example, a cancer of the intestine may have already spread to other areas. At its site of origin, it may be causing an obstruction. Palliative surgery may include a bypass operation to relieve vomiting, pain, and distention of the abdomen. It is always important to balance the risks of an operation against the anticipated benefits. Palliative surgery can help some people live a pain-free, fuller, more active life even if complete cure is not possible.

CASE HISTORY
AN IRRITATING GROWTH

MIRIAM HAS BEEN an avid sun worshiper since she was a teenager, taking any opportunity over the years to maintain a deep tan. Recently, she noticed that whenever she put on her glasses, they rubbed against a small, firm sore on the side of her nose. It annoyed her so much that she decided to see her doctor to have the sore removed.

PERSONAL DETAILS
Name Miriam Saunders
Age 46
Occupation Marketing manager
Family She is recently widowed and has no children. Both her parents are well.

MEDICAL BACKGROUND
Miriam has had only minor disorders, including occasional sinusitis and mild allergic eczema. Her doctor has warned her of the high ultraviolet levels of sunlight in southern California, where she lives, but she has consistently ignored his warnings.

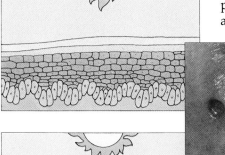

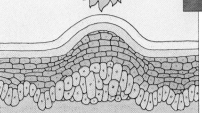

THE CONSULTATION
Miriam tells her doctor that the sore must have been growing slowly for some time. The doctor thinks it might be a harmless sebaceous cyst, but he refers Miriam to a dermatologist to have it checked.

FURTHER INVESTIGATION
The dermatologist asks Miriam about her sunbathing habit. She presses the sore on Miriam's nose and finds it firm, almost hard, and

Sunlight and cancer
Prolonged exposure to the sun carries the risk of skin cancer caused by ultraviolet radiation. Always wear a sunscreen when you expose your skin to strong sunlight.

unyielding. The skin around the sore moves freely over the underlying bone. Under magnification, the dermatologist can see tiny, threadlike blood vessels growing across a rounded edge and a central depression. She decides that a microscope examination of the cells in the sore is necessary.

THE DIAGNOSIS
A plastic surgeon applies a local anesthetic and removes a small sample, from which a thin slice is cut, stained, and mounted on a slide. Under the microscope the cells are revealed to be typical of BASAL CELL CARCINOMA. This type of skin cancer does not spread to other parts of the body, but it does cause local tissue destruction.

THE TREATMENT
Miriam's cancer could be treated effectively with either radiation therapy or surgery. The surgeon tells Miriam that the cancerous growth should be removed and that there will be only a minor scar. The operation is painless and takes half an hour. A deep dime-sized circle of skin surrounding the cancer is excised. After loosening the surrounding skin, the surgeon pulls a small flap across the cavity and stitches the edges together.

THE OUTLOOK
Examination of the removed skin under a microscope confirms that the tumor has not extended below skin level, so there is little danger of a recurrence. After a week the stitches are removed and the scar heals quickly. Aware that she has a higher-than-average chance of another skin cancer, Miriam no longer sunbathes. She uses sunscreen on exposed areas of skin and wears a large hat on sunny days.

SURGICAL PROCEDURES
REMOVAL OF A COLON CANCER

S URGICAL REMOVAL **is frequently a successful treatment for cancer of the colon. The object is to remove the tumor and a wide border of healthy intestine above and below it, along with any lymph glands that may be affected. If possible, the surgeon then rejoins the cut ends of the colon. A typical operation for removing a tumor in the descending colon (on the left-hand side of the body) is shown at right.**

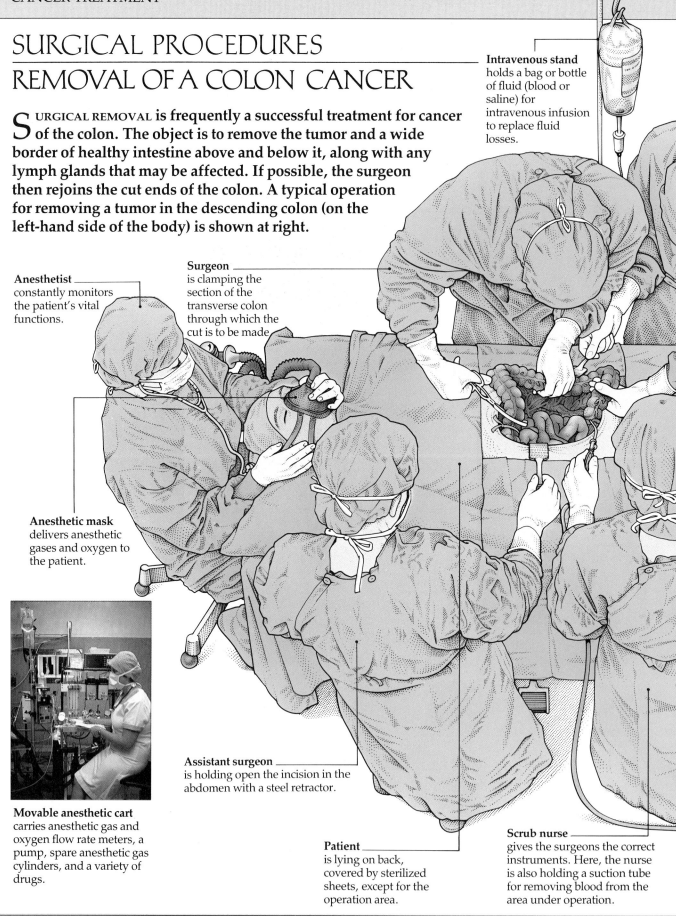

Intravenous stand
holds a bag or bottle of fluid (blood or saline) for intravenous infusion to replace fluid losses.

Anesthetist
constantly monitors the patient's vital functions.

Surgeon
is clamping the section of the transverse colon through which the cut is to be made

Anesthetic mask
delivers anesthetic gases and oxygen to the patient.

Movable anesthetic cart
carries anesthetic gas and oxygen flow rate meters, a pump, spare anesthetic gas cylinders, and a variety of drugs.

Assistant surgeon
is holding open the incision in the abdomen with a steel retractor.

Patient
is lying on back, covered by sterilized sheets, except for the operation area.

Scrub nurse
gives the surgeons the correct instruments. Here, the nurse is also holding a suction tube for removing blood from the area under operation.

1 Cancers of the colon generally develop from small benign masses (adenomatous polyps) that grow into the bowel channel. They may initially cause bleeding. Later, when the tumor has grown, there may be a change of bowel habits, abdominal pain, and obstruction of the intestine. The tumor may invade the bowel wall and spread to nearby lymph glands and other organs.

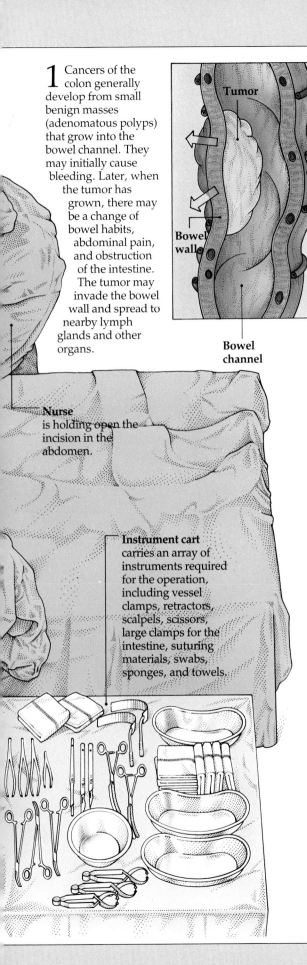

Tumor

Bowel wall

Bowel channel

Nurse
is holding open the incision in the abdomen.

Instrument cart
carries an array of instruments required for the operation, including vessel clamps, retractors, scalpels, scissors, large clamps for the intestine, suturing materials, swabs, sponges, and towels.

2 Preparation for surgery includes the use of enemas, a special diet, and antibiotics taken by mouth; these preparations render the colon as clean as possible. At the start of the operation, a long incision in the middle of the abdomen provides access to the colon. The transverse colon is clamped and tied off at a point well above the site of the cancer.

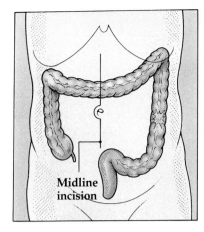

Midline incision

3 Cuts are made in the transverse colon and sigmoid colon to isolate the descending colon. Cuts must also be made in the trunks of the blood and lymphatic vessels that supply the part of the colon to be removed and in the mesentery (the membranous curtain through which the blood vessels travel).

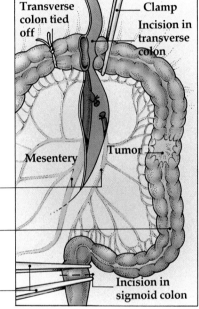

Transverse colon tied off

Clamp

Incision in transverse colon

Mesentery

Tumor

Blood vessels

Descending colon

Clamps

Incision in sigmoid colon

4 After the segment of colon has been removed, the cut ends are rejoined. This is now possible in almost all cases of colon cancer. The rejoining alleviates the need for a colostomy, an operation in which the upper, free end of the colon is brought through the abdominal wall to allow the discharge of feces into a bag worn by the patient.

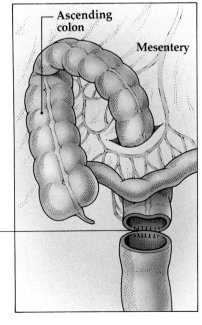

Ascending colon

Mesentery

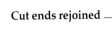

Cut ends rejoined

RADIATION THERAPY

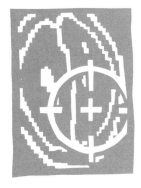

R ADIATION THERAPY is the use of ionizing radiation to treat cancer. The treatment works by changing the structure of the molecules inside normal and cancerous cells, causing a chain of chemical reactions. The most extensive alterations caused by radiation take place in the DNA (genetic material) of the cancer cells. Either the abnormal cells are destroyed completely or their ability to reproduce themselves is reduced, slowing the spread of the cancer.

External radiation
Radiation generated by machines outside the body is known as external radiation. The two brain scans below, obtained by single photon emission computed tomography (SPECT), show the effect of external radiation on a brain tumor. In the upper scan, taken before radiation therapy, the bright area corresponds to blood flowing through the tumor. The lower scan, taken after radiation therapy, shows blood flow has decreased, meaning the tumor has shrunk.

Ionizing radiation is a form of invisible electromagnetic energy. The energy spectrum ranges from longer wavelength, lower-frequency energy, such as radio waves, to very short wavelength, high-frequency energy, such as X-rays and gamma rays. The radiation used in therapy lies at the short wavelength, high-energy end of the spectrum. Although all cells, normal or cancerous, are disrupted by radiation, radiation is most damaging to cells that are dividing rapidly – which is true of most cancer cells. The cancer cells are also less able to

recover from radiation damage, making it possible for repeated small doses of radiation to kill the cells without irreversibly damaging surrounding healthy tissue. Radiation can be used, with or without surgery or chemotherapy, to eliminate certain cancers. It can also destroy the abnormal cells associated with leukemia. Radiation is also used to reduce the size of an advanced tumor to relieve symptoms. Finally, radiation is used to try to destroy any cancerous cells remaining in the body after a tumor has been surgically removed.

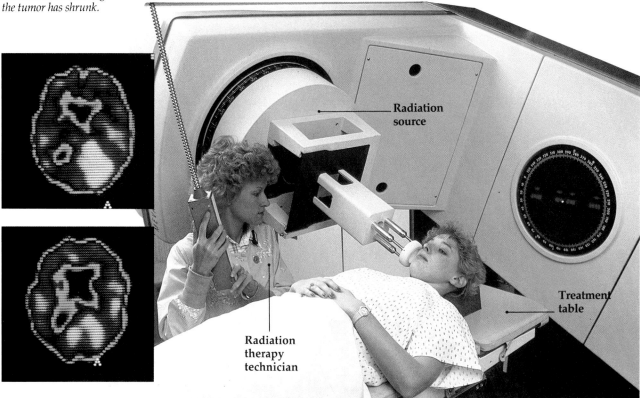

Radiation source

Treatment table

Radiation therapy technician

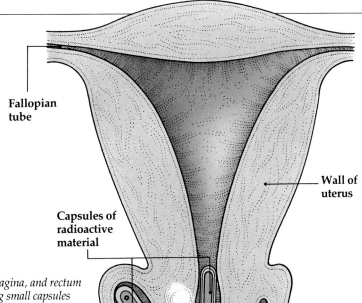

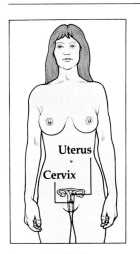

Internal radiation
Cancers of the uterus, cervix, vagina, and rectum are frequently treated by placing small capsules containing radioactive substances such as radium, cobalt, or iridium isotopes directly inside the body cavity near the tumor. The capsules remain in position for a short time, bombarding the tumor with gamma radiation. In the case of cervical cancer (above and above right), sources of radiation may be placed both in the neck of the uterus and in the upper part of the vagina.

Fallopian tube

Capsules of radioactive material

Wall of uterus

Tumor in cervix

Vagina

RECEIVING RADIATION THERAPY

Radiation therapy machines can deliver accurate doses of radiation to any area inside the body. Occasionally, a radioactive source is placed inside the body for a short time to target a very high dose directly onto a cancer.

On the first visit to the radiation therapy department, the radiation oncologist defines the extent of the cancer and uses X-ray images and a simulator machine to plan treatment. The plan depends on the nature and location of the tumor and whether treatment is intended to shrink or eliminate the tumor.

The machines used in radiation therapy are imposing and can be intimidating. However, the size and complexity of the machines is simply a reflection of the energy levels and accuracy demanded of them. The patient lies on a table under a part of the machine while the technologist adjusts the position from the adjoining control room. If the head is to receive therapy, small plastic head gear may be used to make sure that the patient is in exactly the same position for each treatment. Before treatment, the technologist may place custom-made lead shapes on a tray above the patient to shape the radiation field to individual needs.

The radiation dose
The technologist, who can see and talk to the patient from the control room, then begins the treatment, which is usually given in a series of small doses called fractions. The session lasts only a few minutes and the patient experiences no sensation during the treatment. If the patient is receiving radiation therapy from a source inside the body, he or she may stay in the hospital briefly because the radiation could affect other people. Once the radioactive material is removed, the patient goes home.

SIDE EFFECTS OF RADIATION THERAPY

People undergoing radiation therapy should expect side effects, which vary dramatically according to the area of the

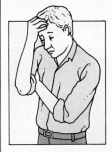
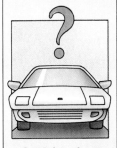

HOW RADIATION THERAPY IS PERFORMED

Radiation therapy is perhaps the most remarkable of all cancer treatments because it harnesses a form of energy that most of us regard as extremely dangerous. Because the types of radiation used affect healthy tissue as well as cancerous tissue, the treatment approach must ensure that maximum damage is caused to the cancerous tissue while minimizing damage to healthy tissue. Each treatment plan must be individually tailored according to the site and extent of the tumor.

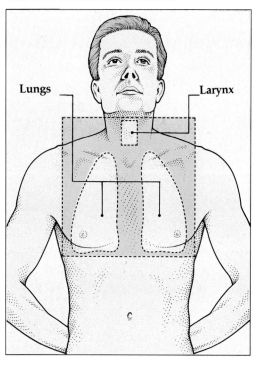

Lungs

Larynx

Radiation source

Lead blocks

Transparent plate

What types of radiation are used?
Today's high-intensity radiation therapy involves either linear accelerators or radio-isotopes (such as cobalt 60) as the radiation source. Linear accelerators are machines that accelerate electrons to a high energy level. The electrons can be used either directly for radiation therapy or to produce high-energy X-rays. Cobalt 60 machines (which are now being phased out) produce gamma rays. The different types of ionizing radiation have varying tissue-penetrating abilities, making them useful for treating tumors of varying extent and depth beneath the body surface.

Radiation beam

Radiation field

Treatment of a wide area
For treatment of extensive malignant tumors, radiation may need to be applied over a wide area, while healthy tissue is shielded from damage. The illustrations above and at right show how radiation is applied over an extensive area to treat cancerous lymph glands in the chest and neck region of a person who has Hodgkin's disease. Custom-made lead blocks attached to a transparent plate between the radiation source and the patient shield the patient's lungs and larynx. A typical treatment schedule consists of daily sessions of several minutes each for about a month. Special care must be taken to position the patient precisely for each treatment.

Rotating radiation source

The source from which the radiation emits can usually be rotated around the treatment table. This allows the patient to remain in one position while the beam is directed at his or her body from different angles. A few centrally located tumors can be for treated by a beam of radiation continuously emitted from a rotating source, as shown at right. Treatment is divided into doses, or fractions, by means of radiation beams aimed at the tumor from different directions (see below).

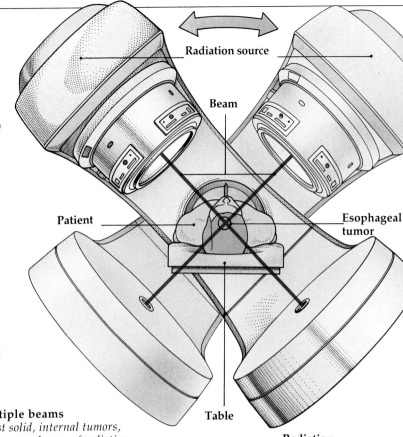

Radiation source

Beam

Patient

Esophageal tumor

Table

Multiple beams

For most solid, internal tumors, relatively narrow beams of radiation are directed at the tumor from several different angles. This ensures that a high dose of radiation is received by the tumor and the adjacent areas of tissue, while much lower doses are received by the surrounding healthy tissues. The diagram below, of a cross section through the chest, shows a three-beam method for irradiating a tumor of the esophagus. The color-coded contours (from yellow, through shades of orange, to red, as calculated by a computer) represent increasing doses of radiation.

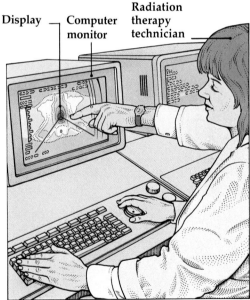

Display

Computer monitor

Radiation therapy technician

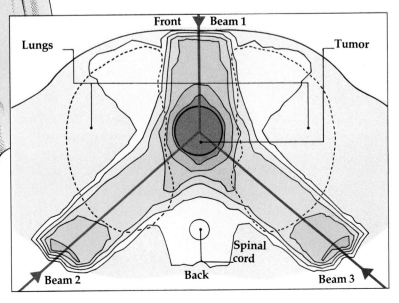

Lungs

Front — Beam 1

Tumor

Spinal cord

Back

Beam 2

Beam 3

Planning treatment

Treatment is often planned using computer simulation. Two- or three-dimensional information about the shape of the patient and the location and size of the tumor (obtained from X-rays and scans) is fed into the computer. The planned paths of radiation through the body are also entered. The contours of radiation intensity in the treatment area are calculated by the computer and displayed on the monitor.

HYPERTHERMIA

Hyperthermia is heat treatment that raises the temperature of a tumor and the area around it by a few degrees. Hyperthermia kills cancer cells, but this treatment is still experimental. Raising the temperature of tumors of the skin or just under the skin by inserting a heat probe into the tumor has been somewhat effective (when used with radiation therapy) in providing palliative treatment to cancers that have not responded to more conventional therapy.

body being treated. Depending on the area and the amount of body tissue being irradiated – especially if large curative doses are used – radiation sickness may gradually develop. Radiation sickness, which may include nausea and vomiting, varies from person to person and dissipates soon after completion of the therapy. Abdominal radiation may cause nausea, vomiting, and diarrhea.

Some treatments cause a sunburnlike reddening or soreness of the skin. Long-term radiation therapy occasionally causes scarring and damage of the irradiated tissues, and there is a small risk of a new cancer developing later. Hair loss is common, but the hair usually begins to grow back after therapy is completed. Finally, ovaries and testes may be rendered sterile by radiation. During pregnancy, treatment should be avoided when possible because of its potentially harmful effects on the fetus.

HOW RADIATION CAN AFFECT THE HEAD

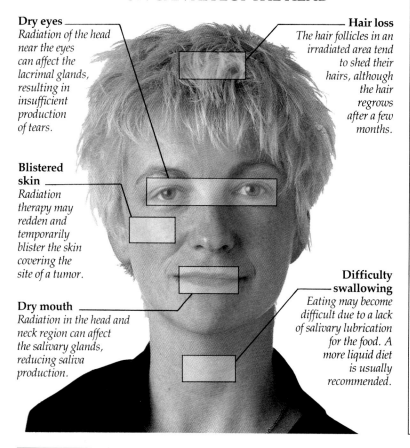

Dry eyes
Radiation of the head near the eyes can affect the lacrimal glands, resulting in insufficient production of tears.

Hair loss
The hair follicles in an irradiated area tend to shed their hairs, although the hair regrows after a few months.

Blistered skin
Radiation therapy may redden and temporarily blister the skin covering the site of a tumor.

Dry mouth
Radiation in the head and neck region can affect the salivary glands, reducing saliva production.

Difficulty swallowing
Eating may become difficult due to a lack of salivary lubrication for the food. A more liquid diet is usually recommended.

ASK YOUR DOCTOR
RADIATION THERAPY

Q **My wife is afraid that her radiation therapy may make her radioactive and potentially harmful to our family. How can I reassure her?**

A No form of radiation administered from outside the body can make her radioactive. If she is receiving internal radiation therapy she will be slightly radioactive for a brief period during hospitalization, but there is no reason to worry once the radiation applicators are removed.

Q **I have been told that I must have radiation therapy after surgery for breast cancer. How bad will the side effects be?**

A Your side effects could be limited to tiredness and slight nausea. The therapy lasts for 4 or 5 weeks (up to 20 visits is common) and most women are able to complete the therapy.

Q **My grandfather is in the hospital with bone cancer and his doctors have chosen radiation therapy to relieve his pain. How does this work?**

A Bone cancers occur inside the bone; as they expand they exert pressure that produces pain. Radiation therapy relieves the pain by reducing the size of the cancerous masses.

Q **Why is my cancer of the larynx going to be treated with radiation rather than by surgical removal?**

A Although radiation and surgery together cure about 90 percent of laryngeal cancers, radiation alone may be preferred at certain stages because surgery frequently produces permanent loss of the voice.

CASE HISTORY
A PERSISTENT SWELLING IN THE NECK

WHEN GREG FIRST DISCOVERED a lump in his neck he knew that it was a swollen lymph gland because he had suffered from mononucleosis as a teenager. He had been feeling sick, had recently lost weight, and had a notable lack of energy and appetite. Suspecting a recurrence of mononucleosis, he made an appointment with his doctor.

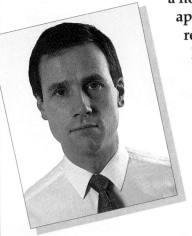

PERSONAL DETAILS
Name Greg Goldin
Age 29
Occupation Computer operator
Family He is single. Both his parents are alive and well.

MEDICAL BACKGROUND
Greg had measles, chickenpox, and mumps as a child, and a severe case of mononucleosis at the age of 18 while he was in college.

THE CONSULTATION
Greg tells his doctor that some weeks ago he had a sore throat and was feverish at night. He had noticed the lump in his neck at that time and, although the sore throat cleared up, the lump persisted. The lump is usually painless, even when pressure is applied, but he has noticed that whenever he drinks alcohol it causes a sharp pain in the area of the lump. His doctor is concerned by the size of the swelling and carefully examines Greg's lymph glands, confirming that one in his neck is definitely abnormal and two others need further examination. His liver and spleen are not enlarged and the results of a blood count and chest X-ray are normal. However, Greg's doctor knows that alcohol-induced pain is a rare but recognized symptom of Hodgkin's disease, a cancer of the lymph tissue. She immediately arranges for Greg to have a biopsy of the enlarged gland.

THE DIAGNOSIS
Greg's lymph gland has an abnormal nodular appearance. A microscope examination reveals that most of the cells in the gland have been replaced by cells of a type characteristic of HODGKIN'S DISEASE. Greg undergoes more tests, including CT scanning and a bone marrow biopsy. The doctor determines that Greg has a very early form of Hodgkin's disease. Greg must have an operation to remove his spleen and any abnormal lymph glands discovered inside his abdomen. Other lymph glands that are under suspicion will later be treated by radiation therapy. There is a strong possibility of a complete cure if treatment begins immediately.

THE TREATMENT
The operation confirms that the cancer is located on both sides of Greg's abdomen, and all the major groups of lymph glands are treated with external megavoltage radiation therapy. Lead shielding blocks are used to protect the areas of his body that do not require irradiation, particularly his lungs. The treatment is given daily, 5 days a week for 4 weeks. Greg's side effects include nausea, slight breathlessness, and a dry cough from a mild radiation-induced inflammation of his lungs.

THE OUTCOME
Greg's cancer was caught early and treated promptly. During a checkup 6 years after treatment his doctor finds him completely free of cancer, and his chances of a recurrence are now remote.

The radiation "field"
Yellow light from the radiation source shows the areas of Greg's upper chest and neck that are to receive radiation; those that will not are protected by lead blocks.

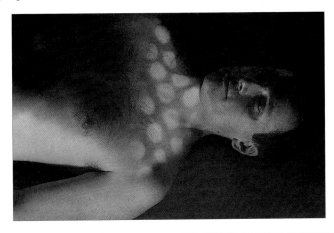

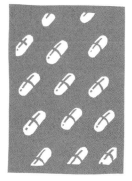

CHEMOTHERAPY

SCIENTISTS HAVE LONG recognized that an ideal cancer treatment would treat the patient's entire body, killing both those cancer cells that have been identified and those that may have traveled through the bloodstream and as yet are undetected. The development of anticancer drugs has made this approach, called chemotherapy, practical in the treatment of a number of cancers.

The use of any drug to treat disease is known as chemotherapy, but the word has come to be associated mainly with anticancer therapy. Most of the anticancer drugs used today work by killing cancer cells. In some cases, such drugs also damage normal cells. The challenge is to maintain the balance between tumor destruction and the toxic effects caused by harming healthy tissue.

CYTOTOXIC DRUGS

The largest group of anticancer drugs are known as cytotoxic drugs because of their cell-killing ability. Although all cytotoxic drugs are capable of killing cancer cells, they work in different ways and can be broadly divided into the categories shown on page 106.

HOW DOES CHEMOTHERAPY WORK?

To be successful, chemotherapy must destroy cancer cells without causing undue damage to healthy tissue. The graph below and the diagrams at right demonstrate the effect of chemotherapy on cancer cells and on bone marrow cells over 16 weeks. Chemotherapy is generally administered at intervals of 3 to 4 weeks to allow healthy tissue (but not cancer cells) to recover between treatments.

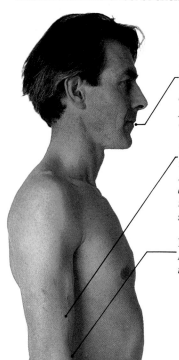

ROUTES OF ADMINISTRATION

Orally
Some drugs are administered orally in the form of syrups, tablets, or capsules.

Subcutaneous injection
A few drugs may be administered by injection into a muscle or under the skin.

Intravenous injection
Many drugs are injected into a vein.

THE CHEMOTHERAPY CYCLE

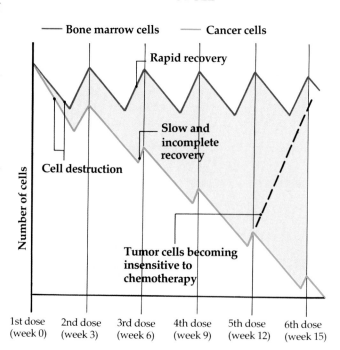

— Bone marrow cells   — Cancer cells

Rapid recovery

Slow and incomplete recovery

Cell destruction

Tumor cells becoming insensitive to chemotherapy

Number of cells

| 1st dose (week 0) | 2nd dose (week 3) | 3rd dose (week 6) | 4th dose (week 9) | 5th dose (week 12) | 6th dose (week 15) |

Cytotoxic drugs cause the most damage to rapidly growing and dividing cells – a characteristic of cancer cells. However, healthy tissues in the body that are constantly reproducing (such as the lining of the gastrointestinal tract and bone marrow cells) are also susceptible to the toxic effects of chemotherapy. Apparently, chemotherapy damages cancer cells preferentially because of the cancer's high growth rate. Also, healthy cells have the ability to repair damage (which may help them recover from any damage done in chemotherapy) but cancer cells may lose that damage-repairing ability through chemotherapy.

The problem of toxicity

The damage caused to healthy tissue during chemotherapy may produce serious side effects during long-term ther-

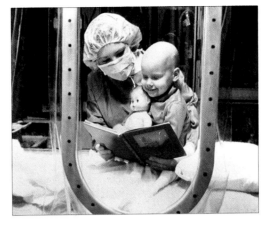

apy. Because cytotoxic drugs interfere with the activity of rapidly dividing cells, they may affect the bone marrow and the intestinal lining, along with the hair follicles and the mouth. Some side effects include suppression of blood cell production, leading to increased susceptibility to infection; anemia and an increased

Weakened immunity
Chemotherapy can weaken the immune system. The drugs may damage the rapidly dividing bone marrow cells, meaning that fewer white blood cells are produced to fight infection. At left, a child undergoing chemotherapy is isolated in a laminar flow chamber (which assures a steady flow of pure air) to prevent exposure to infection.

UNDERSTANDING YOUR TREATMENT

Here is a checklist of questions to ask your doctor if you have been advised to have chemotherapy.

◆ Why is drug treatment necessary?
◆ What are the goals of treatment?
◆ How will the treatment be given, how often, and for how long?
◆ Are any immediate side effects likely?
◆ Are there any long-term side effects?
◆ Where will I get the treatment?
◆ About how long will each treatment take?
◆ After treatment, can I drive home by myself?
◆ Are any special precautions necessary?
◆ What steps should I take to avoid infection?
◆ Are there any symptoms to watch for and under what circumstances should I telephone you?

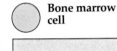

● Cancer cell

○ Bone marrow cell

✸ Cancer cell destroyed or damaged by drug

✷ Bone marrow cell destroyed or damaged by drug

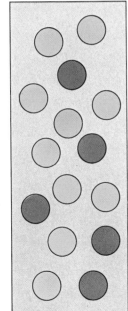

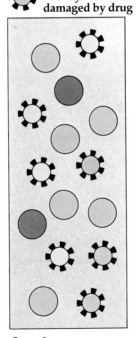

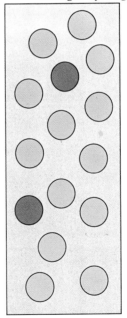

Stage 1
At the outset of treatment, chemotherapy destroys or damages as many bone marrow cells as cancer cells.

Recovery
During the interval between treatments, the bone marrow cells repair themselves and their numbers return to an acceptable level. The cancer cells are slower to recover and reduced in number.

Stage 2
Another dose of chemotherapy causes another reduction in the number of cancer cells and in bone marrow cells.

Recovery
Again the bone marrow cells recover faster. Repeated treatments may lead to a cure unless cancer cells become drug resistant or unless the dosages needed to eliminate all cancer cells prove toxic.

tendency toward bleeding; nausea and vomiting; fatigue; soreness of the mouth; hair loss; and allergic reactions. In addition, certain drugs may damage the kidneys, heart, lungs, liver, and nervous system.

Doctors encourage their patients to consider and accept the possibility of toxic effects if the drug regimen offers a high likelihood of a cure. However, if the disease is incurable and the chemotherapy is being used only to shrink a tumor or improve symptoms, the oncologist recommends using drugs that are less toxic so that the treatment will not do more harm than good. In such cases, the doctor monitors the progress of the cancer and continues the treatment only if there is evidence of benefit to the patient. If all available treatments are too toxic or if the less toxic treatments produce no response, the doctor may recommend supportive care without chemotherapy. Finally, oncologists may also offer the option of experimental treatment.

DRUGS COMMONLY USED TO TREAT CANCER

DRUG TYPE	DRUG NAME
Alkylating agents Drugs that react chemically with DNA.	Busulfan, carmustine, chlorambucil, cisplatin, cyclophosphamide, dacarbazine, lomustine, mechlorethamine, melphalan, semustine, streptozocin, thiotepa
Antibiotics Drugs that have only a weak antibiotic effect but can kill cancer cells.	Bleomycin, dactinomycin, daunorubicin, doxorubicin, mithramycin, mitomycin
Antimetabolites Drugs that interfere with the production of DNA.	Cytarabine, floxuridine, fluorouracil, mercaptopurine, methotrexate, thioguanine
Mitotic inhibitors Drugs that interfere directly with cell division.	Vinblastine, vincristine, vindesine
Other types Drugs that cannot be categorized in the above groups.	Asparaginase, etoposide, hexamethylmelamine, hydroxyurea, procarbazine, mitotane

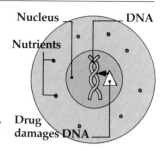

Alkylating agents and cytotoxic antibiotics
These drugs damage the genetic material (DNA) in the cell nucleus, preventing the cell from dividing and growing.

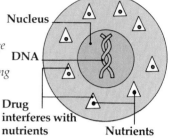

Antimetabolites
These drugs damage cells by preventing them from processing nutrients that are essential to normal growth.

BIOLOGICAL THERAPIES

Scientists have long thought that the body's natural immune defense mechanisms could be manipulated to help control or destroy cancer cells. Recent discoveries have led to the development of "biological" therapies that work on this principle.

Boosting the immune response

Biologists have discovered that interferons, a group of proteins produced naturally by body cells, may be used to increase the activity of T-lymphocyte killer cells (a group of specialized cells that are part of the immune system). Genetic engineers can now make some interferons in the laboratory. Administering doses of an interferon can enhance the ability of the immune system to fight cancer.

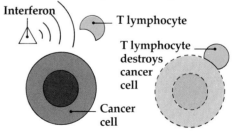

Stimulating the immune system
Raising the level of interferons in the body increases the activity of T-lymphocyte cells, the white blood cells that are capable of attacking and destroying cancer cells.

COPING WITH THE SIDE EFFECTS OF CHEMOTHERAPY

The side effects of chemotherapy vary from drug to drug and from person to person. Patients should ask about the potential side effects of their particular treatment since several drugs are often used together, thus increasing the range of effects. All patients will not suffer all possible side effects of chemotherapy.

SIDE EFFECTS	CAUSES	DRUGS RESPONSIBLE	MINIMIZING THE EFFECTS
Nausea and vomiting	Some drugs irritate the stomach, causing nausea and vomiting. Others act directly on the vomiting center in the brain. Antiemetic drugs can help control these symptoms.	Cisplatin Cyclophosphamide Doxorubicin Fluorouracil Melphalan Mercaptopurine Methotrexate Procarbazine	◆ Eat small meals frequently for a day or so after chemotherapy and avoid drinking large amounts of fluid at one time. ◆ Take any antinausea treatment prescribed, preferably before your first chemotherapy session.
Infection	Infection is the most frequent cause of illness in patients undergoing chemotherapy because the treatment reduces the number of white blood cells being produced by the bone marrow and thus weakens the immune system.	Chlorambucil Cisplatin Cyclophosphamide Doxorubicin Fluorouracil Melphalan Mercaptopurine Methotrexate Procarbazine	◆ Try to avoid exposure to infection, even though most infections in patients with low white blood cell counts come from within the body. ◆ Call your doctor immediately if you are shivering, feverish, or feeling nauseous.
Bleeding and bruising	Chemotherapy may reduce the level of platelets (the cells responsible for blood clotting) in the blood. As a result, patients may bruise or bleed with the slightest injury.	Chlorambucil Cisplatin Cyclophosphamide Doxorubicin Fluorouracil Melphalan Mercaptopurine Methotrexate	◆ Do not take drugs that contain aspirin. They can interfere with the platelets. ◆ Avoid drinking excessive amounts of alcohol. This may lead to inflammation of the mucous membrane lining the stomach and to bleeding if levels of platelets are low.
Hair loss	Because chemotherapy affects the most rapidly dividing cells of the body, the cells of the hair follicles may be damaged, leading to varying degrees of hair loss. The hair of the scalp, the eyelashes, the eyebrows, and occasionally the body hair may be affected.	Cyclophosphamide Doxorubicin Fluorouracil	◆ Although hair loss is normally only temporary, it can cause severe distress. Many patients find that wearing a wig improves morale. The hair sometimes changes color or becomes thicker or curlier when it regrows.

Although interferons are not a miracle cure for cancer, one of them is a very effective treatment for a rare type of leukemia called hairy-cell leukemia; interferons are somewhat useful in the treatment of a variety of other bone marrow malignancies. Some patients with malignant melanoma or adult kidney cancer may also respond to an interferon. The main side effects of interferons are fever and a "flulike" feeling. With the aid of genetic engineering, another product of the immune system, interleukin-2, can be made in the laboratory. Although interleukin-2 initially proved to have major side effects, some good tumor responses were seen – especially in the treatment of adult kidney cancer and malignant melanoma. The severe side effects (due to leakage of fluid from tiny blood vessels in various organs) have been reduced by changes in the way the drug is administered. Today these approaches have a limited application but they are being tested as an adjunct to other treatments.

ASK YOUR DOCTOR
DRUG TREATMENT

Q Is it true that chemotherapy can actually increase the risk of another occurrence of cancer?

A Many anticancer drugs are also carcinogenic. People treated with or cured by certain chemotherapeutic agents do have an increased risk of cancer. The risk may be further increased among those who receive radiation therapy in addition to chemotherapy. The cancers caused by chemotherapy are often leukemias and solid tumors that are resistant to treatment. However, the risk is very small, and the overall assessment is heavily in favor of chemotherapy.

Q Why is it often necessary to use more than one drug in chemotherapy?

A Most chemotherapy uses more than one drug because cancer cells quickly become resistant to a particular drug. If several drugs are used, each drug killing cells by different mechanisms, the likelihood of any resistant cells emerging may be reduced. Using a combination of drugs also helps to reduce the level of toxic effects that might be experienced with higher doses of one drug.

Q What are the risks of undergoing chemotherapy during pregnancy?

A Chemotherapy can seriously damage a fetus. Doctors usually recommend abortion for women who have been treated with anticancer drugs during the first trimester. Women who think they may be pregnant should take a pregnancy test before starting chemotherapy. In selected instances, chemotherapy may be administered in the second or third trimester if no alternative exists.

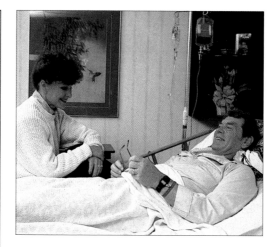

Administering chemotherapy
The picture above shows a patient being given chemotherapy through a vein in the forearm. The procedure is relatively painless.

THE ROLE OF HORMONES

The growth of some cancers is controlled by hormones. Some tumors can be reduced by giving doses of hormones; other tumors respond to drugs that block hormone production.

Breast cancer and prostate cancer are frequently treated with therapy that simulates or opposes the actions of certain sex hormones. If the cancer cells carry receptors for hormones, they often shrink in response to hormone-blocking therapy. This effect is usually temporary but can substantially relieve symptoms. The hormone drugs in use today are:

◆ Tamoxifen – a drug that blocks the effects of the female hormone estrogen. Tamoxifen has been used as a primary treatment for breast cancer, mainly in elderly women; it is used with surgery for other women. Tamoxifen seems to improve chances of survival.

◆ Megestrol – a progestin antagonist.

◆ Progestogens – synthetic forms of the natural female hormone progesterone.

◆ Estrogen – the female hormone.

◆ Androgens – male hormones.

◆ Aminoglutethimide – a drug that blocks the production of the estrogen that is made in the adrenal gland after the menopause.

WHICH CANCERS RESPOND TO CHEMOTHERAPY?

The value of drug therapy varies for different cancers.

Cancers that may be cured by chemotherapy (sometimes with surgery or radiation)

◆ Hodgkin's disease
◆ Non-Hodgkin's lymphoma
◆ Testicular cancer
◆ Choriocarcinoma (tumor of placental tissues)
◆ Acute lymphoblastic leukemia in children
◆ Several rare types of childhood cancers

Cancers in which chemotherapy reduces symptoms and may prolong life

◆ Breast cancer
◆ Small-cell carcinoma of the lung
◆ Ovarian cancer
◆ Cervical cancer
◆ Bladder cancer
◆ Acute leukemia
◆ Myeloma of the bone marrow
◆ Thyroid cancer
◆ Some colon cancers

Cancers that generally respond poorly to chemotherapy

◆ Carcinoma of the lung other than small-cell carcinoma
◆ Primary brain tumors
◆ Malignant melanoma
◆ Kidney cancer in adults
◆ Pancreatic cancer

CASE HISTORY
TESTICULAR CANCER

AFTER READING ABOUT **the importance of testicular self-examination in a magazine, Rod decided to examine his testicles for the first time. He was shocked to discover that his left testicle was larger and harder than his right. He made an appointment to see his doctor immediately.**

PERSONAL DETAILS
Name Rod Jones
Age 29
Occupation Graphic designer
Family No history of any significant disease.

MEDICAL BACKGROUND
Rod has never experienced any serious medical problems.

THE CONSULTATION
After an examination, the doctor confirms that Rod's left testicle is hard, slightly enlarged, and not tender. The doctor refers Rod immediately to a urologist, who orders blood tests and a chest X-ray.

THE DIAGNOSIS
Rod's chest X-ray is normal but a CT scan of his abdomen and chest reveals that the lymph glands at the back of his abdomen are enlarged by a tumor and that he has small cancerous tumors in his lungs. Additionally, the blood test reveals that blood levels of alpha-fetoprotein and human chorionic gonadotropin are raised. These proteins are produced by certain tumors and are usually present with testicular cancer. Rod is told that the enlarged testicle and the raised levels of alpha-fetoprotein and human chorionic gonadotropin indicate that he has TESTICULAR CANCER and that the affected testicle must be removed.

THE TREATMENT
Measurements of alpha-fetoprotein and human chorionic gonadotropin levels taken after the operation show that the levels remain abnormally high, confirming that the cancer has spread to other parts of the body. The doctor recommends chemotherapy and Rod is admitted to the hospital for 5 days. The chemotherapy causes nausea and vomiting, skin problems, and hair loss. Rod returns to the outpatient department on the third and tenth days after his release from the hospital for more chemotherapy. During the treatment, Rod's condition is monitored by measuring the blood levels of alpha-fetoprotein and human chorionic gonadotropin as well as by doing another CT scan after he has had two treatments. These tests show that he is responding well and, after receiving four treatments in all at intervals of one every 3 weeks, he has no evidence of disease.

THE OUTCOME
After his treatment was over, Rod saw his doctor regularly for checkups for several years; there was no sign of a recurrence. Even though Rod had been cured, his doctor told him to continue regular examination of his remaining testicle.

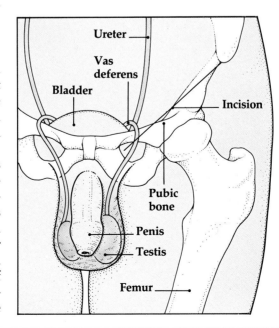

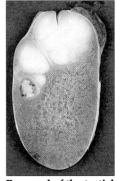

Removal of the testicle
Rod's testicle was removed via an incision in his left groin (see left). The photograph shows a cross section of a testicle that has been removed from the body because of cancer.

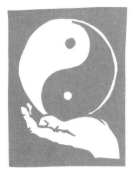

UNCONVENTIONAL TREATMENT

CLAIMS OF MIRACLE CURES for cancer and other diseases are not new; history is littered with false promises made to desperate people. Any such cure should be viewed with extreme skepticism. Some who make these claims are simply "quacks" who are only after money, while others may genuinely believe they can help people. Whichever group a practitioner belongs to, it is important to look at his or her claims objectively.

Unconventional treatment may seem attractive because it provides an opportunity for patients to be active participants in their treatment or because it offers hope when conventional treatment has failed. Some people are attracted to the idea of "natural" treatments. However, turning to untried remedies can lead to more problems, disappointment, and disillusionment.

RELAXATION
Used in conjunction with (and not as a substitute for) conventional treatment, relaxation can help patients cope psychologically and physically with cancer. To start your relaxation session, sit in a comfortable chair in a quiet room with your feet flat on the floor or lie down on a mat. Be aware of the chair or floor supporting your full weight, and pay attention to your breathing, which should be natural and rhythmic. Clear your mind of all thoughts for a few minutes.

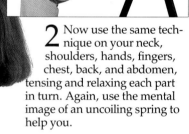

2 Now use the same technique on your neck, shoulders, hands, fingers, chest, back, and abdomen, tensing and relaxing each part in turn. Again, use the mental image of an uncoiling spring to help you.

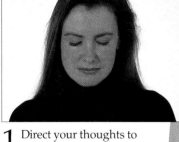

1 Direct your thoughts to your entire face, even your eyes and jaw. Think of an image representing tension, such as a coiled spring. Now imagine the spring unwinding and relax the tension in your face. Tense every muscle in your face and then relax, imagining the spring uncoiling as you do so.

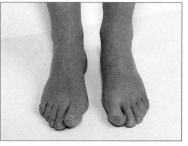

3 Relax your thighs, calves, feet, and toes. Your whole body should now be completely relaxed. Rest quietly. "Bring yourself back" gently and gradually by stretching your arms and legs.

TYPES OF TREATMENT

Many unconventional practitioners offer cancer treatments that may consist of the following.

Visualization, relaxation, and meditation

While there is no evidence that these approaches can kill cancer cells, they may be a useful adjunct to conventional therapy for some people. Some major centers are investigating these techniques further.

The goals of relaxation and meditation are to release muscular tension and achieve a state of mental calm. One relaxation technique is described on the opposite page. Meditation consists of focusing the mind on a single sound, word, or image, or concentrating on the natural rhythm of breathing. Visualization is essentially meditation in which the concentration is directed toward a specific, positive image, such as cancer cells being defeated by white cells.

Relaxation, meditation, and visualization can help patients tolerate the discomforts of cancer and its treatment. Conventional medical practitioners do not disapprove of such approaches because they may help relieve depression, fear, and anxiety. They may also help reduce the nausea and vomiting that can accompany chemotherapy.

Dietary measures

Diets that are used as cancer treatment are usually vegetarian and low in fat. There is no evidence that any diet or particular food can shrink an established cancer. Some people whose tumor is affecting their intestines may find that a high-fiber diet exacerbates symptoms; it can also precipitate bowel obstruction.

Specific remedies

Taking amygdalin (Laetrile) or megadoses of vitamins to cure cancer has received significant media attention.

Amygdalin (Laetrile)
Amygdalin is a preparation that is derived from apricot pits. There is absolutely no evidence to support claims that it is effective in the treatment of any cancer.

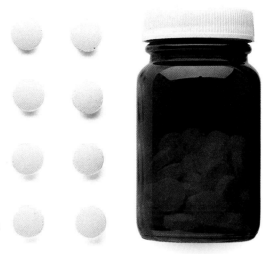

However, clinical trials that have tested the efficacy of amygdalin and vitamin therapies have found them to be completely ineffective. There is no objective scientific evidence that these treatments have a direct effect on cancer.

Some practitioners are involved in dispensing a variety of unproven therapies. Use extreme caution if you are considering unorthodox or unconventional treatment. Ask any alternative practitioner offering cancer remedies to show you research studies substantiating the remedies; also ask how many patients have been treated successfully and unsuccessfully and what kinds of cancer they were treated for. Then ask your doctor what he or she thinks of the treatment.

Detoxification

This form of treatment, which is based on eliminating any possible sources of poison from the body, has a long and checkered past. At one time, medical fashion sanctioned removing a patient's teeth or tonsils, but this approach has long since been abandoned. Similarly, use of coffee enemas as a means of "cleansing" the body has also been totally discredited.

IMPORTANT FACTORS

Some "natural" remedies are said to work only if "unnatural" treatments are abandoned. Never stop potentially curative conventional therapy and do not stop taking drugs that treat symptoms.
◆ Discuss detoxification or other specific remedies with acknowledged cancer experts. Lists of apparent "cures" or individual testimonials are not sufficient evidence of effectiveness.

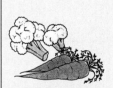

◆ Be careful when choosing special diets. They may result in further weight loss and weakness or make symptoms worse.
◆ If visualization, meditation, and relaxation are offered as the primary (as opposed to supplementary) treatment, be suspicious and ignore claims that you can cure your own cancer if you can perfect the technique.

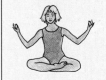

CHAPTER SIX

LIVING WITH CANCER

INTRODUCTION

PSYCHOLOGICAL ASPECTS OF CANCER

TREATING THE SYMPTOMS OF CANCER

EACH GENERATION SEEMS to have an illness that is particularly shrouded in fear and ignorance. Early this century, tuberculosis was the disease that was especially feared. In many of today's motion pictures and TV programs, the heroic figure is dying of cancer. These powerful images have resulted in a variety of misunderstandings about the disease. In the past, the attitude of the medical profession was dramatically different, since doctors (often at the insistence of the patient's family) did not always talk honestly with people in whom cancer had been diagnosed. In many instances, doctors withheld the bad news because they believed that it would maintain hope, sustain the patient, and enable him or her to carry on. However, today doctors agree that a full discussion of a diagnosis of cancer may be more helpful than harmful to the patient. Changing ethical and legal standards have also contributed to this openness about the patient's illness. Patients today are encouraged to ask questions about their illness, and most doctors are willing to answer in as much detail as the patient would like. The supporting role of family members has also been found to be of great value; today, family members are encouraged to participate in discussions about diagnosis and treatment. Revisions in our attitudes toward cancer are not the only changes that have occurred over the last 20 years. There has also been great progress in detection and treatment. Some cancers are curable if they are detected early. Others that may not be curable can be treated, offering the cancer patient many more years of active

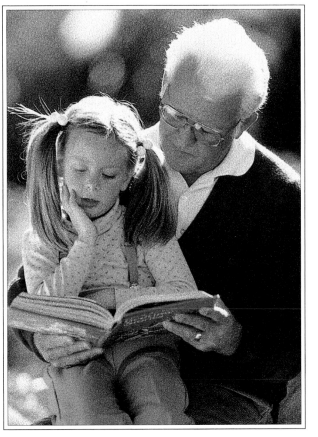

life. Because cancer patients are now living longer, more attention is being paid to their needs after treatment has been completed. Rehabilitation, with the aim of enabling the person to return to as active a life as possible, represents an important part of the total care of the cancer patient.

In spite of the improved prospects, there are still cases where treatment fails and death is inevitable. However, even with terminal cancer, there have been improvements in therapy. Patients need no longer fear that they are destined to die a painful death. Some of the most important breakthroughs in cancer medication have occurred in the area of pain control. With the increasingly sophisticated use of narcotics and other intervention, doctors are now able to assure terminal cancer patients that any pain will be controllable.

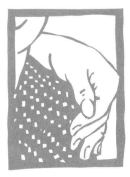

PSYCHOLOGICAL ASPECTS OF CANCER

O VER THE YEARS, cancer has been a subject that many people have been reluctant to discuss. As a result, numerous misunderstandings have arisen. Even today, some people assume that a diagnosis of cancer means inevitable and painful death, and many are surprised by how much progress has been made toward achieving a cure. In the 1990s, there is a greater understanding that life is possible after a diagnosis of cancer.

Good communication is an essential aspect of cancer care. In the past 20 years, it has become commonplace for a doctor to have frank discussions with the patient and his or her family. However, even as recently as the 1960s, many cancer patients were not told of their diagnosis. In addition, family members who were aware of the diagnosis were asked not to discuss it with the patient. Today, the patient and family members can choose to be involved from the time cancer is first suspected, through diagnosis and treatment.

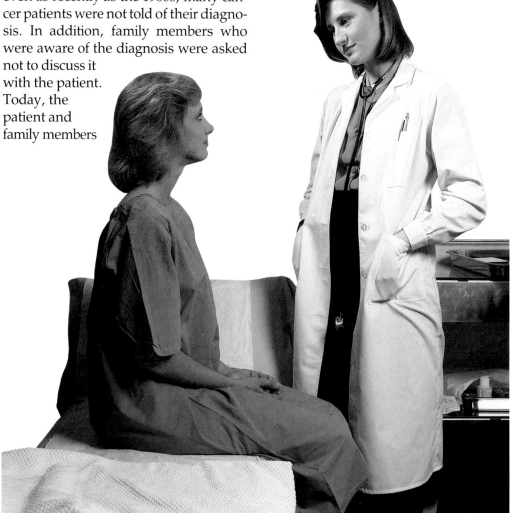

Discussion with the doctor
When a diagnosis of cancer is made, the doctor meets with the patient to explain, as clearly as possible, what treatment is available and what the outlook is. It is usually helpful for a spouse, partner, or close friend to be present during the discussion to help the patient understand and interpret the information. Taking notes while in the doctor's office allows the patient and his or her partner to clarify issues later by phone or during the next office visit.

DETECTION

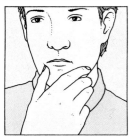

The discovery of a symptom or a lump that may be cancer can be a shock. Studies of psychological reactions to cancer confirm the intense anxiety associated with its discovery. New imaging techniques and simple methods of biopsy (see page 82) have accelerated the process of diagnosis, with results often available within 1 or 2 days. In some areas, though, there can be delays in access to several of these technologies.

A clear explanation

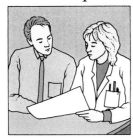

Most patients find it easier to cope if the diagnostic and therapeutic process is explained. If you do not understand what tests or treatments your doctor is recommending, ask questions. Your doctor should be willing to explain his or her procedures.

COPING WITH A DIAGNOSIS OF CANCER

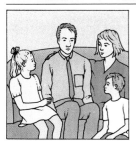

When a diagnosis of cancer is made, the patient and

family should discuss with the doctor all potential treatments. It is difficult to remember every detail about such a conversation – especially if you have just learned you have cancer – so several conversations to

review the same information may be necessary. Again, ask questions. The National Cancer Institute provides a service to inform the public of the availability of treatment trials for a variety of cancers. The time spent by the patient and family discussing with the doctor how they feel about the diagnosis and choices of treatment can do much to reduce anxiety and depression later.

The value of discussion

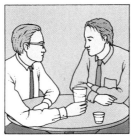

Sometimes, it is useful for the patient to speak to a person removed from his or her family – another doctor, the clergy, or a trusted friend – to attempt to put the situation in perspective. Only rarely do decisions about cancer need to be made on an emergency basis. In most cases, a few days of careful discussion and planning are possible and are almost always worthwhile.

Information brochures
Information is available from a variety of sources that tell you about specific cancers and how they respond to treatment.

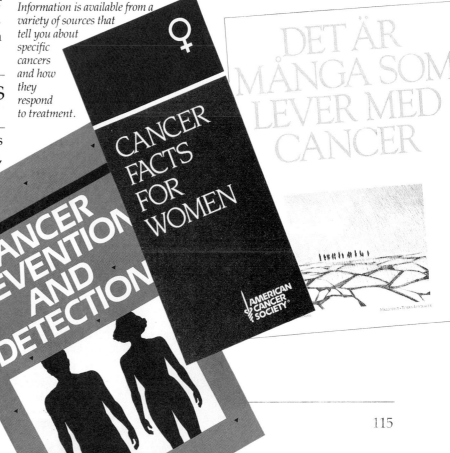

ASK YOUR DOCTOR
LIVING WITH CANCER

Q I have just heard that I have cancer and my instinct is to put the idea completely out of my mind. Am I wrong?

A Not necessarily. But you should be aware of some of the benefits of openly discussing your illness with family, friends, or the clergy. Don't deny yourself an opportunity to come to terms with the facts of your disease. You may find that the facts are much less horrifying than your worst fears.

Q Is my mental attitude likely to affect my chances of recovering from cancer?

A No one can deny the strength of the relationship between mind and body, or that each has an enormous influence on the other. Your state of mind is reflected in many organic changes – muscular tension, heart rate, the output of various hormones, even various immunological changes. These, in turn, can have a bearing on the outcome of any disease.

Q My father, who lives with me, has cancer, and I am told that he does not have long to live. When the time comes, where is the best place for him to die?

A There is no blanket rule for every situation. However, many people feel the best place to die is at home where family and friends are close. There may be practical difficulties but these can often be overcome by visits from nursing and medical staff. If the conditions in your home make this impossible, hospice care is an alternative.

How do people react?

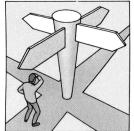

A person may react to the diagnosis of cancer in a number of very different ways, some of which are described below. There is no "correct" response to a cancer diagnosis. A person will respond in a manner that is psychologically appropriate to his or her personality and circumstances. It is helpful to recognize what reactions might occur so that further discussions about the disease can proceed in a direction and at a pace that are best for the patient.

◆ **Denial.** To avoid confronting the situation, some people refuse to believe the diagnosis. Denial may delay treatment and can therefore be destructive. However, an adaptive degree of denial can help patients to live more comfortably with their illness.

◆ **Stoic acceptance.** With this approach, the person acknowledges the diagnosis in a realistic fashion but shows little distress or curiosity. He or she seems resigned to whatever fate will bring.

◆ **Anger.** Some people react with anger and hostility. They feel it is unfair that they have cancer, while others do not.

◆ **Fighting spirit.** Some people view cancer as a challenge to be overcome. These people are eager to participate in decision-making and often develop self-help strategies.

◆ **Helplessness and hopelessness.** In some cases, the person reacts with anxiety and depression; he or she is passive, pessimistic, and feels guilty.

◆ **Playing the sick role.** Those who have spent all their lives taking care of others, sometimes out of a sense of duty (and often without reward), may suddenly find themselves the center of attention for the first time. Without realizing it, they may accept the role of the invalid because they are receiving more attention than they ever had before.

Emotional support
One of the most important ways in which family and friends can help a person with cancer is to provide emotional warmth, support, and understanding.

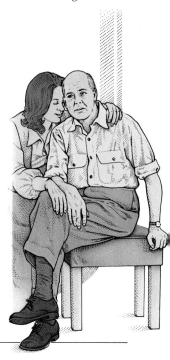

Why me?

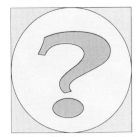

Coming to terms with a potentially fatal illness is extremely difficult. In addition, most of us have little training in counseling the terminally ill. Anger, bitterness, and fear are often the first reactions to a diagnosis of cancer. However, in many cases there is a progression through denial to anger, to depression and, finally, to acceptance. The studies of Elizabeth Kübler-Ross document these distinctive stages.

Often the cancer patient's bitter feelings are not recognized by others. If family and friends do sense the bitterness, they are frequently at a loss as to how best to approach the person. Sometimes, loved ones try to help the patient repress his or her unpleasant emotions and, in doing so, hamper further communication. In other cases, family and friends are afraid to say anything at all about the person's condition. It is important for the patient to be able to express anger, which is a normal and understandable reaction. If the anger is suppressed, it can turn into serious depression. Most people work through their anger and reach a stage of acceptance. They come to realize that, even though their time may be limited, they can make use of the time they have. Sometimes they resolve to enjoy the rest of their life in the fullest possible way.

CANCER INFORMATION SERVICE

A nationwide toll-free telephone service, sponsored by the National Cancer Institute, is available to answer your questions about cancer. The number to call is 1-800-4 CANCER. In Alaska, the number is 1-800-636-6070 and on Oahu, Hawaii, it is 1-800-524-1234 (call collect from neighboring islands).

REHABILITATION AFTER CANCER TREATMENT

Almost all patients who have been treated for cancer need some form of rehabilitation. The type of rehabilitation depends on many factors, including the site and stage of the cancer and the type of treatment that has been performed. The goal is always to allow the patient to return to as normal a life-style as possible. To this end, not only must the physical needs of the patient be attended to, but also his or her psychological, social, and vocational needs. Many rehabilitation programs and self-help organizations have improved the quality of life for cancer patients.

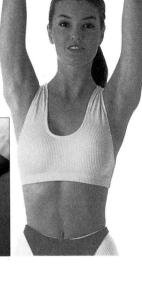

Mastectomy
An increasing number of women who have had a breast removed have the breast reconstructed by means of a skin and muscle graft or a silicone rubber implant (below). The procedure can restore a remarkably normal appearance. After a radical mastectomy, an operation in which lymph glands or muscles have been removed, exercises are needed to maintain shoulder and arm mobility.

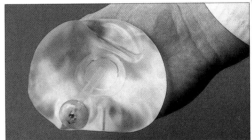

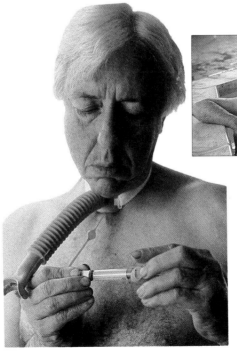

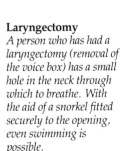

Laryngectomy
A person who has had a laryngectomy (removal of the voice box) has a small hole in the neck through which to breathe. With the aid of a snorkel fitted securely to the opening, even swimming is possible.

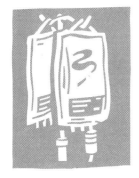

TREATING THE SYMPTOMS OF CANCER

DOCTORS HAVE AN ARSENAL of treatments available to help control symptoms of cancer. In addition, the cancer patient has a variety of options from which to choose to help him or her cope with the physical problems that may arise. Even in situations in which cancer cannot be cured or controlled, techniques are available in most cases to enhance comfort and reduce pain.

Patient-controlled pain relief

This system allows the patient to control the amount of a painkilling, narcotic drug that he or she receives at home. It consists of a narcotic-filled syringe-type injection pump linked with an intravenous line that is positioned in one of the patient's veins. By pressing a button, the patient releases a dose of the drug. More traditional methods of taking drugs by mouth or injection are useful for most patients.

Management of pain with drug therapy allows many cancer patients to live their lives more comfortably. The cancer patient is encouraged to inform his or her doctor about the degree of pain so that appropriate dosages of pain-relieving drugs can be prescribed.

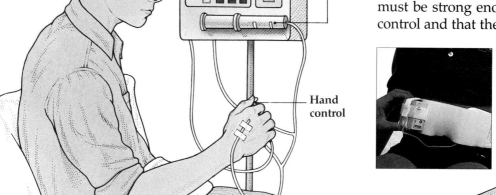

Intravenous line

Injection pump

Hand control

PAIN

Many people associate cancer with pain. They may have seen a relative or friend die in pain or heard of such a situation. In fact, many of the patients who are dying of cancer do not suffer from severe pain. For those who have pain, much can be done to help alleviate it. In every case, a person's emotional state is one of the most important factors in determining his or her perception of pain and how much can be tolerated.

For most patients with incurable cancer, pain-relieving drugs are a mainstay of therapy. The most important principle of pain control is to prevent the onset of pain. This means that a drug dosage must be strong enough to provide pain control and that the drug must be given

Portable pain control
Pain is sometimes controlled by means of a small portable pump strapped to the patient that delivers a narcotic drug continuously into a vein or into the connective tissue under the skin.

often enough so that pain relief is maintained throughout the day. The duration of action of most opiate drugs is about 2 to 4 hours, although preparations of morphine requiring only two or three doses a day are now available. Since pain is influenced by emotion, relieving mood disturbance or sleeplessness often improves pain control. A temporary or permanent nerve block is used to control certain types of pain. Single or continuous pump-controlled injection of narcotics onto the covering surface of the spinal cord is used when almost all other means of pain control have failed. Other pain control methods are applied directly to the central nervous system.

Tolerance to drugs may occur in patients taking narcotics for days or weeks. But this does not necessarily mean pain will re-emerge. The dose can be increased or the drug can be given more frequently. Switching to a different drug is another possible solution.

OTHER METHODS OF PAIN CONTROL

Transcutaneous electrical nerve stimulation (TENS) involves applying minute electrical impulses to the nerve endings that lie beneath the skin above the affected area. Neurostimulators with electrodes that stimulate tracts within the spinal cord or brain have also been employed. In a nerve block, painful sensations are interrupted by injecting a short-acting local anesthetic near the nerve or by using injections that damage the nerve permanently.

OTHER SYMPTOMS

Advanced cancer may be associated with many symptoms other than pain. The following is a short list of some of the more common symptoms.

Nausea and vomiting

Nausea and vomiting can be caused by different mechanisms, some mechanical (such as obstruction of the upper gastrointestinal tract) and others indirect (such as increased pressure on the brain). Other causes of nausea are the pain itself, pain medication, high blood calcium levels, a peptic ulcer, or chemotherapy. In these cases, the symptoms are treated by correcting the underlying disorder if possible. When the nausea has no obvious cause, treatment may include antiemetic drugs. If vomiting is persistent, an intravenous infusion of fluid while the patient temporarily stops eating and drinking may help.

CARE AT HOME
◆ Avoid any foods that make you nauseous ◆ Eat little and often ◆ Avoid large volumes of fluids ◆ Follow advice on medication

Constipation

Strong painkillers can cause constipation. Weakness, reduced mobility, poor fluid intake, a diet low in fiber, and depression also contribute. Often, a stool softener, a tap-water enema, or a stimulant laxative is prescribed. However, daily use of suppositories may be all that is required. A 6-ounce glass of prune juice each day may also be helpful.

CARE AT HOME
◆ Be sure your diet contains fruits, vegetables, oatmeal, and stewed prunes. Also, six to eight glasses of water every day will help you pass stools that are not hard or dry.

PAINKILLERS USED IN CANCER TREATMENT

Pain medications can be grouped according to strength. The doctor usually starts at the mild end of this scale and increases the dose or strength of the painkiller as required by the severity of the pain. The patient's response helps the doctor decide the amount of the drug needed to control his or her pain.

Nonnarcotic (mild pain)	Mild narcotic (moderate pain)	Strong narcotic (severe pain)
Acetaminophen Aspirin Nonsteroidal anti-inflammatory drugs (NSAIDs)	Codeine Pentazocine Propoxyphene	Hydromorphone Meperidine Morphine Oxycodone

Cough

Coughing may occur as a direct result of cancer or because an infection has developed. If ridding the lungs of phlegm is likely to improve the patient's condition (such as in cases of pneumonia), ample fluid intake will encourage a "productive" cough. If the patient has a dry, irritating cough, which can cause chest pain, drugs such as codeine and dextromethorphan can be helpful. Bronchodilators and expectorants are prescribed for asthmalike symptoms.

CARE AT HOME
◆ Use a humidifier
◆ Do not smoke
◆ Stay warm

Difficulty breathing

Difficulty breathing may develop for a number of reasons. Severe anemia, which can cause breathing problems, is treated by a blood transfusion; pleural effusion (a collection of fluid around the lung) is sometimes treated by inserting a needle through the chest wall and withdrawing the fluid. In other cases, such as a nontreatable lung cancer, oxygen is given to help the patient breathe. Drugs, such as morphine or antianxiety drugs, may also make breathing more comfortable. Drugs that are inhaled can also help.

CARE AT HOME
◆ Call your doctor immediately if severe breathlessness occurs

Insomnia

Pain relief, antidepressants, antianxiety drugs, and sedatives can help insomnia due to pain, frequency of urination, depression, fear, and night sweats.

CARE AT HOME
◆ Try to maintain a normal nighttime sleeping pattern by avoiding too much daytime sleeping

THE CANCER PATIENT'S DIET

Cancer patients who have poor appetites should eat numerous small meals or snacks rather than three large meals per day. The diet should be rich in protein and high-calorie foods. Some people require liquid food supplements. Vitamins may also be helpful. Special diets are sometimes needed. A clear liquid diet may be given to patients just after an operation; a semi-liquid diet consisting of mashed or pureed foods may be needed for patients who have difficulty swallowing.

HOSPICE CARE

Modern hospices were developed in England in the late 1960s as an alternative to hospital care for people in the last stages of a terminal illness. The first hospice in the US was established in 1974. The hospice team includes doctors and specially trained nurses who are skilled in the management of pain and other symptoms of terminal disease. With other team members, they also provide emotional support and understanding for patients and their families.

Over the past few years the emphasis in some areas has moved away from admission to a hospice and been replaced with hospice-type care in the patient's home. As people lose their fear of cancer, the dignity of dying at home appeals to many.

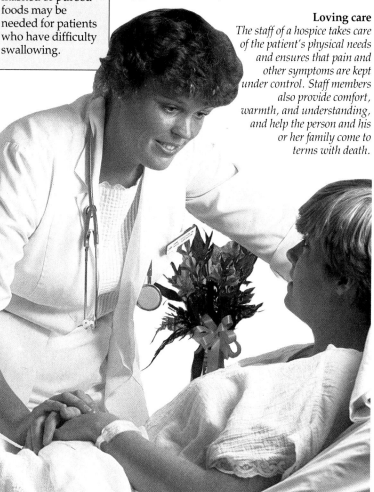

Loving care
The staff of a hospice takes care of the patient's physical needs and ensures that pain and other symptoms are kept under control. Staff members also provide comfort, warmth, and understanding, and help the person and his or her family come to terms with death.

CASE HISTORY
AN INCURABLE CANCER

S ARAH WAS NOTICEABLY **losing weight. Even more upsetting was her obvious loss of appetite and uncharacteristic loss of energy. One day, her husband Don came home from work and found Sarah vomiting. He became alarmed and insisted that she consult their doctor.**

PERSONAL DETAILS
Name Sarah Friedberg
Age 53
Occupation Homemaker
Family Mother died of cancer. Father is well.

MEDICAL BACKGROUND
Sarah has been a three-pack-a-day smoker for many years.

THE CONSULTATION
Sarah tells her doctor that her weakness has been getting worse. She has had moderate pain in the upper part of her abdomen for months and often feels pain in her back now, too. She has not told her family or sought medical help because she has not wanted to worry them. The doctor is concerned to see that the whites of Sarah's eyes have a yellow cast and that her skin has an olive-colored tint. These signs are an indication of jaundice caused by obstruction to the outflow of bile from her liver.

FURTHER INVESTIGATION AND DIAGNOSIS
Ultrasound examination shows a mass high in Sarah's abdomen. She has an operation, which reveals a large PANCREATIC CANCER. The tumor cannot be removed, but the surgeon relieves the obstruction, which eases Sarah's vomiting and the jaundice.

THE OUTLOOK
Sarah's surgeon tells Sarah and Don that the disease is incurable. He explains that, in advanced cancer of the pancreas, treatment can relieve symptoms but that there is no chance of a cure. He also tells them that a variety of investigative studies involving radiation and chemotherapy are being conducted at cancer centers throughout the country under the auspices of the National Cancer Institute. Despite the fact that surgery will not cure the cancer, these programs offer the possibility of a prolonged survival and relief of symptoms. The studies also contribute to knowledge that may ultimately lead to a cure.

The news of Sarah's condition is devastating to her family. Sarah returns home with an attitude that is almost the same as it was before she saw her doctor – one of denial. Some family members deal with Sarah's illness by ignoring it, believing that not discussing it will help alleviate Sarah's anxiety. But Don is convinced that it isn't the most productive approach for Sarah.

THE SEQUEL
One day, Sarah suggests to Don that they should quit pretending. She talks to her children and her sister and encourages them to speak honestly, to express their true feelings, and to grieve together in her presence. Sarah, in coming to terms with her illness, tells her family that she wishes to be with them at home when she dies. Her family accepts her decision. With the help of her doctor and the medical staff who visit her at home, Sarah's last days are filled with warmth and the fond recollections of her loved ones.

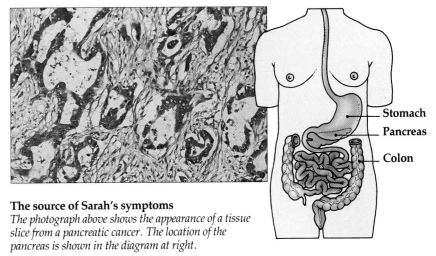

Stomach
Pancreas
Colon

The source of Sarah's symptoms
The photograph above shows the appearance of a tissue slice from a pancreatic cancer. The location of the pancreas is shown in the diagram at right.

CANCER FACT FILE

This section contains information regarding some 30 different types of cancer. They are arranged in order of decreasing incidence, beginning with the most common and ending with some of the most rare. For each cancer, the estimated annual US totals of new cases and deaths from the cancer are given for 1990, along with the incidence (the number of new cases per 100,000 people). For most cancers, the 5-year survival rate – the number of persons with a cancer who are alive 5 years after diagnosis – is stated. Also given are an indication of how the cancer responds to treatment, the age range during which a cancer is most likely to strike, and the factors that may influence its occurrence.

LUNG CANCER

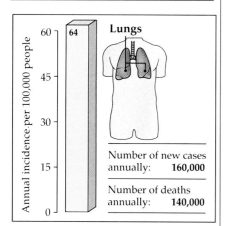

Number of new cases annually: **160,000**

Number of deaths annually: **140,000**

Lung cancer causes more fatalities than any other cancer in the US – about 140,000 deaths a year. It accounts for only 15 percent of all the cancers that occur, but it causes 25 percent of all deaths from cancer because it is so often incurable. Today more men than women get lung cancer because 30 or 40 years ago more men than women smoked. However, the difference in incidence is narrowing and will continue to narrow because more women have been smoking since the 1940s. Blacks have a higher incidence than whites. The majority of cases occur in those 35 to 75, with the highest incidence occurring between the ages of 55 and 65.

Causes and risk factors
At least 85 percent of all lung cancers are attributable to cigarette smoking. The longer the history of smoking and the greater the number of cigarettes smoked, the greater the risk. People who smoke filtered, low-tar cigarettes may be at a slightly lower risk, though the risk is still far higher than that for nonsmokers. Involuntary, or "passive," inhaling of smoke from the cigarettes of other people may also increase the risk. The risk begins to drop as soon as exposure ceases – that is, when you and/or the people around you quit smoking. After about 10 years, the risk drops almost to the level of nonsmokers.

Other risk factors that act in combination with cigarette smoking include exposure to certain industrial substances, such as asbestos, and exposure to radon, lead, chromium, and cadmium. People living in cities have a higher incidence of lung cancer than people who live in the country.

Types and development
There are four main types of lung cancer. One of these is small-cell (oat cell) carcinoma, which accounts for 20 percent of all lung cancers. The three other types are known as non-small-cell carcino-

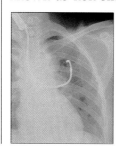

Bronchoscopy
Bronchoscopy sometimes allows lung cancer to be detected. In this X-ray, the tip of the endoscope is visible in the upper part of the left lung.

mas. The differences between the non-small-cell carcinomas are largely outweighed by their similarities. The three types are squamous cell carcinoma, which accounts for about 40 percent of lung cancers and occurs near the center of the chest; adenocarcinoma, which accounts for about 25 percent, tends to occur toward the outside edge of the lungs, and is twice as common in women; and large-cell carcinoma, which accounts for about 15 percent. The reason that lung cancer is so often lethal is that it is rarely diagnosed at an early, treatable stage; usually the disease has spread beyond the lungs by the time it is recognized.

Signs and symptoms
Symptoms often do not appear until the disease is advanced. Warning signals include a persistent cough, sometimes producing sputum streaked with blood, shortness of breath, hoarseness, chest pain, or a persistent chest infection.

Diagnosis
Diagnostic tests include analysis of chest X-ray films and of sputum; computed tomography (CT) scanning; a very thin needle biopsy of a nodule taken through the chest wall; and bronchoscopy (the use of a narrow fiberoptic viewing instrument to examine the airways). A biopsy or brushing of the airway lining for cells may be performed during bronchoscopy.

Treatment

Treatment depends on the type and stage of the cancer. In small-cell cancer, surgery has largely been replaced by chemotherapy – either on its own or with radiation therapy. In cases of non-small-cell disease, surgery, radiation therapy, or chemotherapy are options. Surgery is usually used to treat cancers that have not spread. When lymph glands are affected, surgery may be combined with radiation therapy. In some cases, chemotherapy is also used. When surgery is not possible, radiation therapy and chemotherapy are the mainstays of therapy.

Outlook

Only 13 percent of all patients diagnosed with lung cancer live for 5 years or longer. However, the 5-year survival rate ranges from 33 percent to about 80 percent for cases

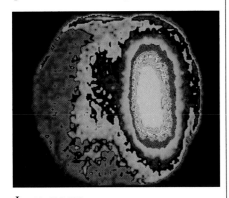

Lung cancer
This color-enhanced radionuclide scan shows a cancer of the right lung (on the left of the image). The uniform colors on the left side indicate that ventilation has ceased due to blockage by a tumor.

detected before they have spread. New approaches, which combine chemotherapy with radiation and surgery, may improve survival for many patients who have operable cancer. The addition of chemotherapy to radiation may help some patients with inoperable cancer. Quitting smoking has the greatest impact on lowering the risk of lung cancer.

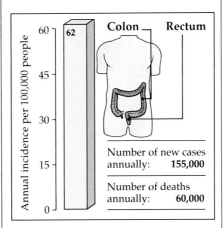

COLORECTAL CANCER

Annual incidence per 100,000 people

Colon — Rectum

62

Number of new cases annually: **155,000**

Number of deaths annually: **60,000**

Like cancer of the lung, cancer of the colon and rectum is a major public health problem in the US. Although there are almost as many cases of colorectal cancer found each year as there are of lung cancer, there are less than half as many deaths from colorectal cancer.

About two thirds of colorectal cancers occur in the colon; one third occur in the rectum. The incidence is approximately the same in men and women, but slightly higher among black males. It is rare before age 50, with a peak in incidence between 70 and 80. There are significant variations within the US; colorectal cancer is common in the northeastern states and less so in the southern and southwestern states. Worldwide, it is more common in developed countries and less so in developing countries.

Causes and risk factors

Some circumstantial evidence suggests that colorectal cancer may be linked with a diet that is high in animal fats and meat and low in fiber. Risk factors for colorectal cancer include a personal or a family history of colorectal cancer, inflammatory bowel disease, colonic polyps, or ovarian or breast cancer. Pelvic radiation therapy also increases the risk.

Types and development

Colorectal cancers start as growths in the inner lining of the bowel, but they may then penetrate the bowel wall and invade other nearby organs. The slow growth of most colorectal tumors and the high diagnostic sensitivity of X-ray and endoscopic examinations often make it possible to detect these cancers at an early stage.

Symptoms and signs

Colorectal cancer has the most favorable prognosis (forecast) when it is identified while it is still localized. Usually, the diagnosis of asymptomatic (causing no symptoms) colorectal cancer is made because a rectal examination reveals a tumor, or an examination of the stools shows chemical evidence of small amounts of blood. The most common symptom of colorectal cancer is bleeding from the rectum. The blood may appear dark or bright red and may streak the stool or be mixed in with it. Other symptoms include a persistent change in bowel habits, a change in the character of the stool, or abdominal pain.

Diagnosis

Two tests are recommended to detect colorectal cancer. The first test, which should be performed annually from about age 40, consists of a digital rectal examination (a test of the feces for hidden blood should be done starting at about age 50). The second test is a visual examination of the rectum and lower colon using a special viewing instrument (proctosigmoidoscopy). This should be done every 3 to 5 years after age 50. People who have risk factors may require more frequent examinations of the lower bowel with an endoscope.

Treatment

Surgery, which is performed via an incision in the abdomen, is the most effective treatment for co-lorectal cancer that has not spread. After surgical removal of the affected section of bowel, the cut ends are rejoined whenever possible. Today, doctors can use stapling devices to reattach the cut ends, which means that the construction of a permanent abdominal opening of the colon (a colostomy) for the elimination of feces is used less often than it once was. In about 15 percent of cases, when the cancer is very low in the rectum (near the anus), a colostomy is required.

The use of a combination of anticancer drugs in addition to surgery has been shown to reduce the rate of recurrence in some patients whose colorectal cancers upon removal have been found to extend to neighboring lymph glands. Radiation therapy with chemotherapy and surgery is sometimes used in cases of rectal cancer.

Outlook
The 5-year survival rate is about 50 percent. If the cancer is detected at an early stage, before it has penetrated through the bowel wall or spread to any nearby lymph glands, the survival rate may be as high as 90 percent. Once a colon cancer has penetrated the bowel wall, survival rates drop to 60 to 80 percent. When lymph glands are affected, the survival rate drops to 30 to 50 percent.

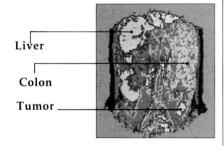

Cancer of the colon
This color-enhanced scan obtained by magnetic resonance imaging (MRI) shows cancer of the colon (the isolated white area at bottom right). The cancer has spread to the liver, which appears massively enlarged at the top and left.

BREAST CANCER

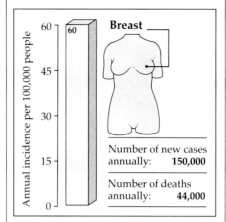

Annual incidence per 100,000 people

Breast

Number of new cases annually: **150,000**

Number of deaths annually: **44,000**

Breast cancer is the most common cancer in American women. It accounts for 27 percent of the cancers that occur in women and its incidence is gradually increasing. White women have a slightly higher incidence than black women. In those parts of the world where the incidence of breast cancer is high, such as the US, Canada, western Europe, and Australia, the greatest risk is after age 65.

Causes and risk factors
Increasing age is a risk factor. Few cases of breast cancer occur before age 30 and most occur after age 50. A family history of breast cancer is a risk factor, though only about 25 percent of women who get breast cancer have a history of it in their family. A woman who has never had a child is at an increased risk, as is a woman who has her first child after age 30. Also significant is the interval between the onset of menstruation and the woman's first full-term pregnancy. A woman who begins menstruating early and who has her first full-term pregnancy after the age of 30, for example, may be at a higher risk. In addition, it is thought that women who have undergone radiation therapy earlier in life and women who experience a late menopause may also be at a higher risk.

Types and development
Breast cancer can affect one or both breasts. Most breast cancers are of a type called adenocarcinoma, which arises from glandular tissue. About 90 percent arise from the milk ducts in the breast, and the remaining 10 percent from the milk-producing breast lobules. There are different subvariations of each of these types, and they vary in their response to treatment. Most cases start as a single lump. The cancer may spread to the lymph glands in the armpit before spreading to the rest of the body.

Symptoms and signs
In addition to a lump in the breast, symptoms may also include changes in the breasts, such as swelling, thickening, dimpling, or skin irritation. Tenderness and retraction of, or discharge from, the nipple may be related to a more advanced stage.

Diagnosis
Any new lump that can be felt in the breast should be suspected as being cancerous, though most are not. In fact, about four out of every five prove to be benign. The American Cancer Society recommends that women age 20 and over perform a monthly breast self-examination. A definite diagnosis can be established only by biopsy. The chances of detecting breast cancer at an early, curable stage have been greatly improved by the introduction of mammography (low-dose X-ray examination), which can locate cancers that are too small to be felt by even the most practiced examiner. It is recommended that women have a mammogram every 2 years between the ages of 40 and 50, and annually after 50.

Treatment
There are several possible approaches to treatment, which can range from lumpectomy (removal

of only the tumor) to various types of mastectomy (see SURGERY FOR BREAST CANCER on page 92), radiation therapy, chemotherapy, and drugs that manipulate hormone levels. The choice depends on the type and stage of the cancer, the woman's age, and her preference. Two or more methods are often used simultaneously. New techniques have made possible breast reconstruction, which is an important part of rehabilitation. In recent years there has been a move toward greater recognition of the emotional consequences of breast cancer. Today, doctors are more aware of the patient's concerns about surgery and possible disfigurement. In addition, self-help groups provide women with a forum for discussion and support.

Outlook

The 5-year survival rate for breast cancer ranges from 90 percent if the cancer is removed at the earliest stage, to as low as 10 percent if it has spread to other parts of the body at the time of diagnosis.

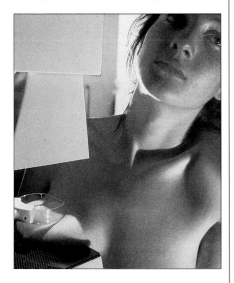

Breast X-ray examination
In mammography, a breast X-ray examination, the breast is gently compressed between two plastic plates and exposed to a low-dose beam of X-rays. The technique allows breast cancer to be detected at an early stage.

PROSTATE CANCER

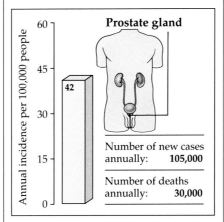

Prostate gland

Annual incidence per 100,000 people

60

45

30

15

0

42

Number of new cases annually: **105,000**

Number of deaths annually: **30,000**

Prostate cancer is, with lung cancer, one of the two most common cancers in American men. Black Americans have the highest incidence of prostate cancer in the world, for reasons that are not fully understood. Worldwide, the incidence is highest in northwestern Europe and North America and very low in Japan.

Causes and risk factors

The incidence of prostate cancer increases with age, with about 80 percent of cases diagnosed in men over the age of 56. There is some evidence that a predisposition to prostate cancer may occur among members of the same family. Workers who are exposed to cadmium are at slightly higher risk. Prostate cancer is one of the few cancers for which no association with smoking has been found.

Types and development

Prostate cancer is, in general, slow growing; it is diagnosed in 65 percent of cases while still localized within the gland. In other cases, the cancer spreads aggressively into adjacent tissues or to other organs.

Symptoms and signs

Patients with highly localized prostate cancer frequently have no symptoms. A diagnosis may be sus-pected during a digital rectal examination. Symptoms, if any, may include a weak or interrupted flow of urine, difficulty starting or stopping urination, pain when urinating, and frequent urination, especially at night. Advanced cancer may spread to bones, causing pain and fractures.

Diagnosis

Men over age 40 should be alert to disturbances in their pattern of urination and should have a digital rectal examination as part of their regular physical examination. Using ultrasound to view the prostate is a new technique being investigated to evaluate whether the cancer is confined to the gland or has spread to adjacent tissue.

Treatment

Surgery or radiation therapy may be used if the cancer is found early. Removal of all or part of the prostate gland is usually performed when the cancer is causing obstruction to the flow of urine. If the cancer is widespread, manipulation of male hormone levels by removal of the testicles or administration of female hormones may relieve pain for long periods by shrinking the tumor.

Outlook

If prostate cancer is diagnosed and treated while still localized within the substance of the prostate gland, about 80 percent of patients live for 5 years or longer. If the tumor has broken through the wall of the gland, the survival rate drops to 60 percent. If the lymph glands are also affected, the survival rate 5 years after treatment is between 50 and 55 percent. Impotence was once a major drawback of the removal of the prostate. However, the development of surgical procedures that spare the nerves controlling erection now prevents impotence in 70 percent of cases.

BLADDER CANCER

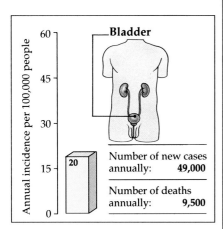

Annual incidence per 100,000 people

Bladder

20

Number of new cases annually: **49,000**

Number of deaths annually: **9,500**

Three times as many men as women are affected by bladder cancer, and the incidence is gradually increasing. Overall, the incidence is higher in urban than in rural areas.

Causes and risk factors
The risk of bladder cancer increases with age, with most cases occurring over age 60. Cigarette smoking is the greatest risk factor; smokers have twice the risk of nonsmokers. Smoking may be involved in causing as many as half of all bladder cancer deaths. Workers in the rubber and leather industries are also at high risk.

Types and development
Bladder cancers vary from small polyps of low malignancy in the surface lining of the bladder to highly malignant tumors that may invade the bladder wall and spread to other organs.

Symptoms and signs
There are no signs or symptoms unique to bladder cancer. The most common signs are blood in the urine, which occurs in 75 percent of cases, and persistent mild irritation when urinating, which occurs in 30 percent of cases. In advanced stages, there may be pelvic pain, rectal obstruction, and swelling in the lower part of the abdomen.

Cancer cells are usually not detected during examination of the urine, but a microscopic amount of blood in the urine may be found. There are, however, many other causes of blood in the urine and full investigation is needed to identify the cause.

Diagnosis
Diagnosis may include examination of the bladder wall with a cystoscope (a slender viewing tube) fitted with a lens and light, which can be inserted into the urinary tract through the urethra. The diagnosis is confirmed by taking a biopsy specimen via the cystoscope.

Treatment
Treatment depends on how advanced the cancer is. Surgery, alone or with radiation or chemotherapy, is used in most cases. If the tumor is still in its early stages, it is usually cut out or treated by diathermy (heat destruction) via the cystoscope. Bladder tumors commonly recur and may be treated with surgery or chemotherapy.

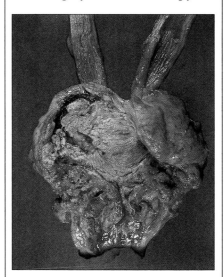

Bladder cancer
This specimen of a cancerous bladder shows a large tumor (gray area). The ureters (tubes that drain the kidney into the bladder) are widened because of the obstruction to the flow of urine caused by the tumor.

Outlook
Almost 90 percent of patients whose bladder cancers are diagnosed at a very early stage live for 5 years or more. If the cancer is more advanced and has spread into or beyond the bladder wall, the 5-year survival rate drops to about 20 to 50 percent.

UTERINE CANCER

Uterine cancers include cancers of the endometrium (lining of the uterus) and cancers of the cervix (neck of the uterus).

ENDOMETRIAL CANCER

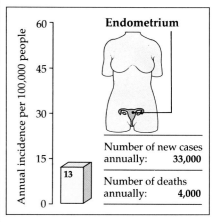

Annual incidence per 100,000 people

Endometrium

13

Number of new cases annually: **33,000**

Number of deaths annually: **4,000**

The incidence of endometrial cancer is increasing in several countries, especially the US. White women have about twice the incidence of black women. The average age at diagnosis is about 60.

Causes and risk factors
Hormone replacement therapy with estrogens alone (which was used until the mid-1970s) has been found to be a risk factor for endometrial cancer. This risk is not incurred when women take estrogen combined with the hormone progesterone as hormone replacement therapy for the treatment of symptoms associated with the menopause. Obesity and starting the menopause after age 52 may increase the risk.

Types and development

Endometrial cancer starts in the lining of the uterus. It may then spread into the cervix (neck of the uterus). The cancer may also penetrate the uterine wall and spread to the fallopian tubes and ovaries and elsewhere in the pelvis and abdomen. In later stages it may spread to other organs, such as the lungs. This cancer is thought to usually have its onset between 55 and 60.

Symptoms and signs

Vaginal bleeding is an early symptom of endometrial cancer. Any bleeding that occurs after the menopause should be reported to your doctor. In advanced stages there may be an increase in the amount of blood and there may be pain with the bleeding. It is recommended that a woman receiving hormone treatment have an endometrial biopsy periodically.

Diagnosis

A Pap smear may suggest a diagnosis of endometrial cancer, although only when the tumor has reached the opening of the cervix (where the Pap smear is taken). A diagnosis can be confirmed only by an endometrial biopsy, a dilation and curettage (D and C), or a hysteroscopy (direct inspection of the uterus) with a biopsy.

Treatment

The usual procedure for endometrial cancer is a hysterectomy (removal of the uterus), oophorectomy (removal of one or both ovaries), and removal of any affected lymph glands. More surgery may be required if the cancer has spread.

Outlook

The 5-year survival rate for endometrial cancer is 80 percent overall, but ranges from less than 25 percent for advanced cases to more than 90 percent for cases in which the cancer has not spread.

CERVICAL CANCER

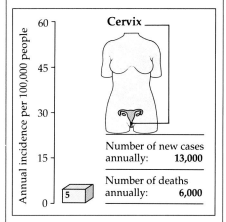

Cervix

Annual incidence per 100,000 people

60

45

30

15

0

Number of new cases annually: **13,000**

Number of deaths annually: **6,000**

5

Cervical cancer is one of the few cancers that can be detected, and often cured, at an early stage. The average age at diagnosis for carcinoma in situ – an early stage in which individual cells of the cervix are malignant but the cancer has not begun to spread – is 25 to 40 years. The average age at diagnosis for invasive (spreading) cervical cancer is between 48 and 55.

Causes and risk factors

A low socioeconomic level, poor hygiene, and having sexual intercourse for the first time in early adolescence place a woman at increased risk of cervical cancer. The risk increases with the number of sexual partners the woman has had and with the number her male partners have had.

Types and development

The cancer can spread from the cervix into the pelvic wall, the parametrium (the ligaments and tissues supporting the cervix and uterus), and the vagina. It may block the ureters, which carry urine from the kidneys to the bladder. Advanced cancer may spread to the bladder and the rectum.

Symptoms and signs

Symptoms and signs of cervical cancer depend upon the stage of the disease. At a preinvasive stage, there are usually no symptoms. In an early invasive stage, there may be vaginal discharge and bleeding, and some spotting or bleeding after sexual intercourse. During the later stages, there may be a bloody discharge, pelvic pain, pain in the upper back parts of the legs, and frequent urination.

Diagnosis

If precancerous or malignant cells are found in a Pap smear, the Pap test may be repeated. If the test result is positive, the cervix is examined with a colposcope (a viewing instrument) and a biopsy may be performed.

Treatment

Precancerous areas that have been detected are treated by removal of the affected area by cryotherapy (treatment with extreme cold) or laser. If there is any evidence that the cancer has become invasive, the uterus is removed. For tumors that involve deeper layers of the uterus, a radical hysterectomy (which includes removal of regional lymph glands), or radiation therapy, is performed.

Outlook

The 5-year survival rate for cervical cancer is 66 percent overall, but ranges from about 10 percent in advanced cases to 90 percent if it is discovered in the early stages.

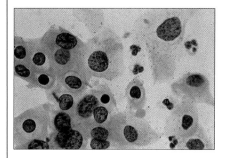

Abnormal cervical (Pap) smear
This microscope view of cervical cells shows precancerous changes. The abnormal cells have large, dark nuclei.

LYMPHOMAS

Lymphomas are cancers of lymphatic tissue. They are classified by their appearance when seen under a microscope. The most common type of lymphoma in young people is Hodgkin's disease. All the other lymphatic tissue malignancies are known as non-Hodgkin's lymphomas. These lymphomas differ significantly from Hodgkin's disease. In addition, they vary greatly from one type to another in their growth patterns and response to therapy.

HODGKIN'S DISEASE

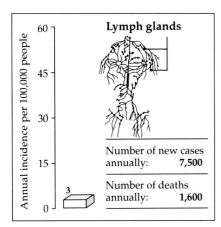

Hodgkin's disease (sometimes referred to as Hodgkin's lymphoma) is a cancer of the lymph glands that mostly affects people in their early 20s. It also occurs frequently in the elderly. Few cases of Hodgkin's disease are found in the age groups in between. There is a higher incidence of Hodgkin's disease in men than women.

Causes and risk factors

The unusual age peaks in the distribution of the disease have suggested many theories about the cause of Hodgkin's disease, but the actual causes and risk factors remain unknown.

Types and development

Hodgkin's disease often seems to start in the lymph glands that are located in the neck and chest region. The disease then may progress to affect the lymph glands or organs below the chest. In some cases, an exploratory abdominal operation may be required to determine if the disease has spread below the chest.

Symptoms and signs

Hodgkin's disease causes painless swelling of the lymph glands, often in the neck, chest, or abdomen. Patients are considered to have a more advanced form of the disease if they have fever or sweating or if they have lost more than 10 percent of their body weight.

Diagnosis

Positive diagnosis is made by lymph gland biopsy and examination of the biopsy sample under a microscope by a pathologist.

Treatment

Radiation therapy alone can be used to treat patients whose disease is located only in the chest and neck. In more widespread disease, radiation therapy is used in conjunction with a combination of anticancer drugs.

Outlook

The treatment of Hodgkin's disease is one of the major success stories of modern cancer therapy.

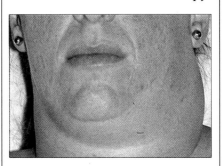

Hodgkin's disease
This woman's enlarged neck is the result of swelling of lymph glands due to Hodgkin's disease (a type of lymphatic cancer).

Today few patients whose conditions are diagnosed at a reasonably early stage, and who are properly treated, die of the disease. The 5-year survival rate for all cases of Hodgkin's disease is more than 70 percent. For people whose disease is confined to a single site at the time of diagnosis, the survival rate is more than 90 percent.

NON-HODGKIN'S LYMPHOMAS

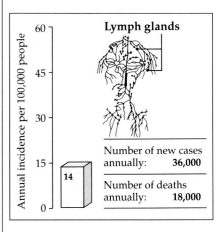

These cancers are the sixth most common cause of death from cancer in the US and are increasing in incidence. The average age at diagnosis is 42. Non-Hodgkin's lymphomas affect males slightly more often than females and white people more often than black.

Causes and risk factors

The causes are unknown but some forms, such as Burkitt's lymphoma, are clearly related to infection with the Epstein-Barr virus. Lymphomas are much more common in people who have weakened immune systems, such as people with AIDS, than in those with healthy immune systems.

Types and development

The non-Hodgkin's lymphomas fall into several different categories, depending on the type of cells of the lymphatic system that have been transformed into cancer cells and the pattern these cells form under a microscope. The non-Hodgkin's lymphomas vary widely in the rate at which they grow and spread and the effects they produce. Some of these cancers grow and spread rapidly and may require aggressive therapy. Others wax and wane for months or years without requiring any therapy.

Symptoms and signs
A non-Hodgkin's lymphoma may begin as a painless enlargement of lymph glands. The disease may affect a wide variety of organs, from the brain to the gastrointestinal tract. As with Hodgkin's disease, there may be loss of weight, fever, and sweating. In some people, the disease produces a greater-than-normal susceptibility to a variety of infections.

Diagnosis
A positive diagnosis is made by removing one of the enlarged lymph glands for examination. Highly sophisticated laboratory methods are needed to identify precisely the type of cell that has become malignant. Sometimes the doctor must open the chest or abdomen to obtain an affected gland or organ.

Treatment
Treatment varies with the type and extent of the lymphoma. Some slow-growing lymphomas may not require therapy for months or years. Other rapidly growing and spreading forms may require chemotherapy consisting of combinations of potent anticancer drugs. In some cases radiation therapy alone may be effective. In other cases, radiation therapy may be given in addition to chemotherapy.

Outlook
The outlook varies with the type of non-Hodgkin's lymphoma, but the overall 5-year survival rate is at least 50 percent.

ORAL CANCERS

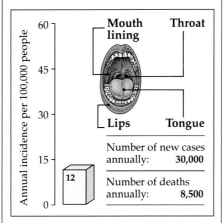

Cancers of the head and neck include those that affect the lips, mouth, tongue, and throat. For most of these cancers, the usual age at diagnosis is over 40. In the US, the incidence is four times as high in males as in females.

Causes and risk factors
The most significant risk factor is the use of tobacco – including cigarettes, pipes, cigars, and chewing tobacco. The site of an oral cancer often corresponds directly to the site of tobacco exposure, such as where the tip of a pipe makes contact with the mouth or where a plug of chewing tobacco is held between the cheek and gums.

Alcohol is strongly associated with cancer of the mouth, especially when it is used along with tobacco. A person who drinks 1.5 ounces of alcohol and smokes 40 or more cigarettes every day has 15 times the risk of a person who neither drinks nor smokes. Poorly fitting dentures and broken teeth may also increase the risk of mouth cancers.

Types and development
Cancer can develop in any part of the oral cavity, including the lips, gums, floor and roof of the mouth, tongue, tonsils, salivary glands, and back of the throat (pharynx).

Symptoms and signs
Early warning signs include a sore in the mouth that bleeds easily and does not heal, a lump or thickening, or a persistent red or white patch. Late changes include difficulty or painful chewing, swallowing, or moving the tongue or jaw.

Diagnosis
Doctors diagnose cancers of the mouth and throat by performing a biopsy of the suspicious area. Parts of the mouth that are difficult to see directly can be investigated with the help of special mirrored tools or fiberoptic instruments.

Treatment
Radiation therapy and surgery have been the standard treatments for oral cancers that have not spread. Chemotherapy is being studied as an addition to surgery and radiation therapy in some cases. Radical face and neck surgery is required to treat oral cancers that are more advanced. However, such surgery has a deforming effect on the face and neck. Major advances have been made in reconstructive surgery and prosthetics to help restore the appearance.

Outlook
The 5-year survival rate is about 50 percent overall. However, it ranges from more than 90 percent for lip cancer to about 30 percent for cancer of the throat.

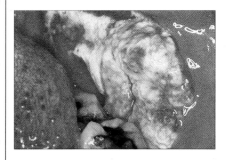

Mouth cancer
Cancer of the mucous membrane that lines the cheek is visible in patches within the white, lumpy area.

LEUKEMIA

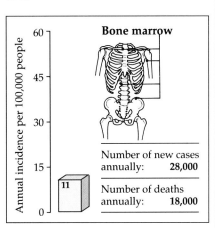

Bone marrow

Annual incidence per 100,000 people

Number of new cases
annually: **28,000**

Number of deaths
annually: **18,000**

Leukemia is a cancer that is characterized by the proliferation of abnormal white blood cells in the affected person's bone marrow (where all blood cells originate).

Types and development
Leukemia is classified into several different types according to the class of white cell that has been affected. Untreated, the so-called acute leukemias are rapidly fatal diseases. Acute lymphocytic (or lymphoblastic) leukemia is the most common type in children. Among adults, acute myelogenous leukemia is the most common acute leukemia. It is slightly more common in men than women and its incidence is markedly increased in both sexes after age 65. Overall, about 75 percent of cases of acute leukemia occur in adults; about 8 percent occur in children, but leukemia is still the most common cancer in childhood.

In contrast to the acute leukemias are chronic myelogenous leukemia and chronic lymphocytic leukemia. The chronic leukemias usually occur in middle age or later and tend to run a slower course.

Causes and risk factors
The causes of leukemia are largely unknown. However, several risk factors have been identified. Acute leukemia is 20 times more common in people with Down's syndrome and 40 times more common in the identical twin of a person who has leukemia than it is in the general population. It is much more common in a child whose mother was exposed to radiation early in pregnancy. Any form of ionizing radiation, including X-rays, can cause leukemia. Many more cases than normal occurred in Hiroshima and Nagasaki in the 20 years following the nuclear explosions.

Other risk factors include exposure to chemicals such as benzene and arsenic, and many of the drugs used in cancer chemotherapy.

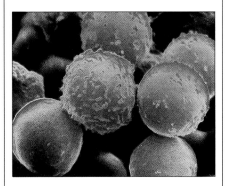

Leukemia
This color-enhanced image taken with an electron microscope shows immature and abnormal white cells in a blood sample taken from a patient with acute lympho-blastic leukemia.

Symptoms and signs
In acute leukemia, the overgrowth of abnormal white cells tends to crowd out production of the oxygen-carrying red cells and of normal white cells and platelets (cells involved in blood clotting). Depletion of the red cells results in severe anemia. Although white cells may be present in excess, they are abnormal and unable to perform their usual function of defending the body against infection. This leads to multiple infections. Loss of platelets may interfere seriously with blood clotting and lead to bleeding. The symptoms of chronic leukemia develop much more slowly. Symptoms such as a persistent raised temperature and night sweats may develop in addition to symptoms common to the acute leukemias.

Diagnosis
In some cases the diagnosis can be made by a routine blood count, which usually includes a white cell count. The white cell count can be raised by infections, but the count is rarely raised to the levels found in leukemia. A blood test may also reveal the type of cell present. However, a bone marrow aspiration (in which marrow is removed from the bone) and a biopsy confirm the diagnosis and determine the type of leukemia.

Treatment
The different forms of leukemia call for different kinds of highly sophisticated treatment, most often using anticancer drugs in different combinations. Sometimes chemotherapy is combined with radiation therapy. Surgery is rarely used in the treatment of leukemia, except for removal of the spleen, which is performed in cases of a rare form of the disease – hairy-cell leukemia. For all leukemias,

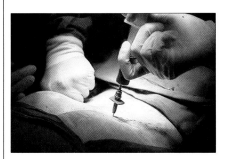

Bone marrow transplant for leukemia
Leukemia may be treated by destroying abnormal bone marrow and replacing it with healthy marrow from a donor (if a donor with compatible marrow can be found). Healthy bone marrow is sucked out through a needle from the donor's hipbone (as shown here). It is then injected into the recipient's bloodstream, which carries it to the bones.

supportive measures such as transfusion of red cells, white cells, and platelets can be helpful. Whole body radiation and/or massive chemotherapy treatments with subsequent bone marrow transplantation can be used for some forms.

Outlook

The overall mortality of acute leukemias in adults is about 80 percent; the survival rate is much better – over 50 percent – for acute lymphoblastic leukemia in childhood. The long-term survival rate for chronic myelogenous leukemia is very low, though the length of the illness varies. A 50 percent cure rate is achieved when massive chemotherapy and radiation therapy is performed with bone marrow transplantation. Treatment for chronic lymphocytic leukemia can prolong life for many years.

PANCREATIC CANCER

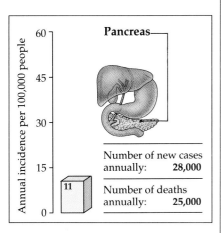

Pancreatic cancer has a very high mortality. The incidence of this cancer is higher in men than in women and the peak age of incidence is between 70 and 79.

Causes and risk factors

Smoking is a major risk factor. The incidence in heavy smokers is double that in nonsmokers. Chronic inflammation of the pancreas, es-

pecially in people who drink heavily, is probably also a risk factor.

Types and development

Very few pancreatic cancers originate in the insulin-producing or other endocrine cells of the pancreas. Most cancers arise in the glandular tissue that secretes, or the ductal tissue that delivers, digestive enzymes into the duodenum. Pancreatic cancer is usually diagnosed at an incurable stage.

Symptoms and signs

Cancer of the pancreas is insidious, causing few or no symptoms in the early stages. When symptoms do occur, they may include abdominal pain, sometimes radiating to the back, loss of appetite, and loss of weight. Though the affected person may feel no pain, jaundice and itching (caused by blockage of the ducts that carry bile from the liver) often occurs when the cancer involves the head of the pancreas.

Diagnosis

Diagnosis is frequently difficult. CT scanning, MRI, or ultrasound scanning may show a mass in the region of the pancreas. A needle biopsy can often help diagnose the disease. However, an exploratory operation may be necessary.

Treatment

If the cancer has spread, surgery may help as a palliative (symptom-relieving) measure. Connecting the gallbladder to the intestine allows the tumor blockage to be bypassed and helps relieve jaundice and itching. Pancreatic cancer responds poorly both to radiation therapy and chemotherapy.

Outlook

About 90 percent of people who have pancreatic cancer die within a year of diagnosis regardless of treatment.

SKIN CANCER

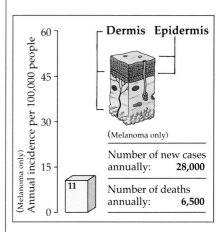

Skin cancers fall into two groups. The first includes nonmelanomas (basal cell carcinomas and squamous cell carcinomas), which are usually not serious and can be treated easily. The second group includes the malignant melanomas, which are much more dangerous. Any skin cancer, however, can be fatal if ignored and not treated. Nonmelanomatous skin cancers are very common and doctors believe they are grossly underreported. It is estimated that more than half a million cases of nonmelanomatous skin cancer occur each year in the US. Malignant melanomas are much less common but the incidence is increasing.

Causes and risk factors

The incidence of nonmelanomatous skin cancer is directly proportional to the degree of exposure to ultraviolet light, the most common source of which is sunlight. Because sunlamps and tanning salons also deliver ultraviolet light, they pose risks as well. People with fair skin who regularly expose themselves to the sun, especially without protection, are more susceptible to skin cancer.

Malignant melanoma is less strongly related to ultraviolet light exposure, but severe sunburns increase the risk.

Types and development

Basal cell carcinomas spread locally and can cause considerable tissue destruction. Squamous cell carcinomas, although much less common, can also destroy tissue locally and spread widely from their point of origin. Malignant melanomas spread quickly to nearby lymph glands and to other parts of the body.

Symptoms and signs

Basal cell carcinomas are typically raised, hard-edged, and often dimpled in the center. They are pearly colored and shiny, with faint tiny red blood vessels showing on the surface. Squamous cell carcinomas are flatter, more irregular, crusty, and ulcerating. Malignant melanomas are dark, irregularly colored, irregularly shaped tumors that bleed easily and may be ulcerated, tender, scaly, or flaky. Any mole or molelike mark on the skin that undergoes a change in size, configuration, or color should be checked by a doctor.

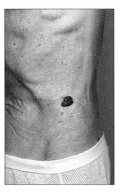

Skin cancer
The brown, raised mark on this man's left side is a malignant melanoma. It is the least common but most serious form of skin cancer.

Diagnosis

Because skin cancers are so easy to see, they can often be diagnosed immediately by a doctor. However, a biopsy should be performed to confirm the diagnosis before treatment is started.

Treatment

Nonmelanomatous skin cancers respond extremely well to treatment, especially if it is provided early. A variety of treatment methods may be used, depending on the type of skin cancer and its location and size. Surgical removal, radiation therapy, electrocautery, freezing (cryosurgery), chemical destruction, or direct application of anticancer drugs may be used.

The treatment of malignant melanoma is more difficult and crucial. When it is discovered early, an attempt is made to surgically remove the entire tumor along with a segment of surrounding tissue. The nearby lymph glands are also examined and may be treated. More advanced melanomas are treated by surgery, radiation therapy, and chemotherapy. Immunotherapy has also been tried.

Outlook

For nonmelanomatous skin cancers the outlook is excellent. For melanomas, the outlook depends on the tumor's location and thickness (depth into the layers of the skin) at the time of treatment. People who have melanomas that have not spread deeply have a 5-year survival rate of 95 percent. Those with deeper tumors have a 5-year survival rate of about 30 to 40 percent.

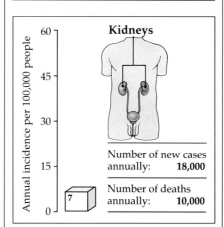

KIDNEY CANCER

Kidneys

Annual incidence per 100,000 people

60
45
30
15
0

Number of new cases annually: **18,000**

Number of deaths annually: **10,000**

7

Kidney cancer is moderately common. Twice as many men as women are affected by this cancer.

Causes and risk factors

Some of the carcinogens in cigarette smoke are absorbed from the lungs into the bloodstream and are excreted in the urine. As a result, kidney cancer is two to three times more likely to develop in cigarette smokers than it is in nonsmokers. Certain industrial chemicals may cause kidney cancer. Some researchers believe there is an association between obesity and kidney cancer in women.

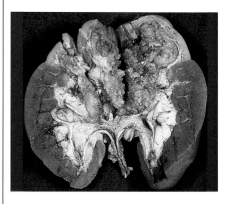

Kidney cancer
This kidney has been cut in half to reveal a large cancerous mass (top, middle area).

Types and development

Most kidney cancers in adults are of the type known as renal cell carcinoma (also called hypernephroma), which usually occurs after age 40. This kidney cancer arises from the cells that line the kidney tubules. Renal cell carcinoma may spread rapidly, often infiltrating the veins of the kidneys and spreading along them. The cancer may also spread via the bloodstream to the lungs, bones, liver, and other organs.

Another type of cancer, called nephroblastoma or Wilms' tumor, occurs in children and accounts for a significant percentage of all childhood cancers. Most cases of Wilms' tumor are discovered before the age of 3 years. This tumor also can grow rapidly and can spread to the lungs, liver, and brain. Survival has improved in recent years.

Symptoms and signs

The principal sign of kidney cancer is blood in the urine, which occurs in about half the cases. A dull pain and local swelling in the back are less common and usually occur only when the tumor has reached a considerable size. Fever, loss of weight, loss of appetite, and weakness are common.

Diagnosis

Kidney cancers are most often detected by X-ray imaging or by ultrasound scanning. The X-ray imaging techniques used involve introducing a radiopaque contrast medium (dye) either into the urinary tract (as in pyelography) or into the blood supply to the kidneys (as in renal angiography). A CT scan and MRI may also be used to evaluate the extent of the disease. A biopsy is required to confirm the diagnosis. The doctor then makes an evaluation of the tumor's spread into nearby lymph glands and other organs.

Treatment

When only one kidney is affected, it is usually removed, sometimes along with the ureter that services it. If both kidneys are involved, the goal of surgery is to remove all cancerous growth while conserving as much normal kidney tissue as possible. In some cases it is necessary to remove both kidneys. In these cases, the patient must undergo a kidney transplant or regularly have hemodialysis, in which the waste products in the blood are filtered out.

Outlook

The overall 5-year survival rate is 30 to 50 percent. For a tumor that is confined to the kidney and treated by surgery, the 5-year survival rate is about 60 percent. The outlook for children with Wilms' tumor is better; up to 80 percent survive if their treatment begins early.

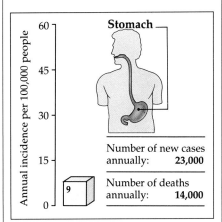

STOMACH CANCER

| Number of new cases annually: | **23,000** |
| Number of deaths annually: | **14,000** |

Stomach cancer has become substantially less common this century. The reasons for this decline are uncertain. The incidence of stomach cancer is higher in men than in women and is most common between 50 and 59.

Causes and risk factors

The causes are not clear, but some researchers believe that dietary factors play a role. Nitrosamines, formed in the stomach from nitrate preservatives in food, are suspected of being involved, as are alcohol and cigarette smoking. Stomach cancer may run in some families, which may indicate a genetic predisposition or nothing more than a sharing of environmental risks, such as eating, drinking, and smoking patterns.

Types and development

Stomach cancer affects the inner lining of the stomach, either in ulcerated, scattered areas or in the form of a polyplike growth. Stomach cancers that have not spread are confined to the stomach's mucous lining and, if ulcerated, may cause pain or bleeding.

Symptoms and signs

The early symptoms of stomach cancer are vague and the sufferer may be unaware that he or she has the disease. Symptoms may be as insignificant as minor discomfort in the abdomen, some loss of appetite, and loss of weight. Later, as the tumor grows, the symptoms become more conspicuous and include a feeling of fullness before completing a meal, difficulty swallowing, pain, nausea, difficulty keeping food down, or blood in the stools. In an advanced case of stomach cancer, a mass may be felt in the upper part of the abdomen.

Diagnosis

If stomach cancer is suspected after special barium X-rays are performed, an examination using an endoscope (flexible viewing tube) is done. A biopsy may be taken, which may provide a firm diagnosis. However, an operation is often necessary to ascertain the extent of the tumor and thus the chances of cure. It is common to find that the tumor is very far advanced.

Treatment

Depending on the location of a tumor in the stomach, either a portion of the stomach or the entire stomach is removed (gastrectomy). Radiation therapy and chemotherapy have been used in various combinations, but the results have not been encouraging.

Outlook

Depending upon the stage of the disease, the 5-year survival rate for people who have stomach cancer ranges from 5 to 85 percent.

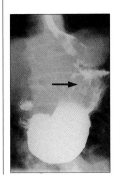

Stomach cancer
This X-ray picture, taken after the patient swallowed a barium solution, shows a tumor (arrow) occupying the entire upper part of the stomach.

OVARIAN CANCER

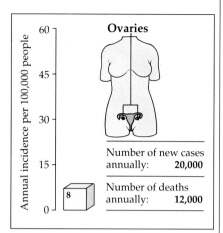

Annual incidence per 100,000 people

Ovaries

Number of new cases annually: **20,000**

Number of deaths annually: **12,000**

Ovarian cancer is responsible for more than half of all deaths due to cancers of the female genital organs. Worldwide, the incidence of ovarian cancer is higher in North America and northern Europe, and lower in Asia and Africa.

Causes and risk factors
The risk for ovarian cancer increases with age, with the highest rates in women between the ages of 65 and 84. Women who have never had children are at twice the risk of those who have had children. The more children a woman has had, the lower the risk. Breastfeeding and the use of oral contraceptives also appear to lower the risk. A history of ovarian cancer in a sister or mother increases the risk, as does a history of breast or endometrial cancer, or cancer of the colon or rectum.

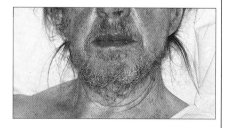

Hirsutism
Some rare forms of ovarian cancer result in hirsutism (excessive hairiness) because the tumor produces excess amounts of male sex hormones.

Types and development
The cancer may be confined to one or both ovaries or may extend to the fallopian tubes, uterus, and surrounding pelvic or other tissues. Extensive spread can involve other abdominal organs. Blood-borne spread of cancer cells may lead to the appearance of secondary tumors (metastases), most often in the lungs or bones.

Symptoms and signs
Ovarian cancer is a "silent cancer" and often shows no symptoms or signs until late in its development. The most common sign is an enlarged abdomen, caused by a collection of fluid. Vague and persistent abdominal troubles, such as discomfort, swelling, pain, or flatulence, may be caused by the tumor pressing against the bowel or bladder. Vaginal bleeding occurs in only 15 percent of the cases.

Diagnosis
Ovarian cancer is best detected by periodic pelvic examinations and ultrasound follow-up evaluation when an ovary is suspected of being enlarged.

Treatment
Treatment includes surgery and chemotherapy. Major inroads against this disease have been achieved through chemotherapy. Surgery usually involves the removal of one or both ovaries, the uterus, and the fallopian tubes. Operations in which as much of the tumor as possible is removed are thought to aid chemotherapy. If cancer is detected early, only the affected ovary is removed.

Outlook
If ovarian cancer is diagnosed and treated early, about 80 percent of patients live for 5 years or longer. When it is diagnosed at an advanced stage, the 5-year survival rate drops to about 25 percent.

BRAIN AND NERVOUS SYSTEM CANCERS

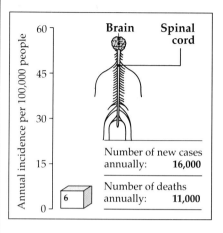

Annual incidence per 100,000 people

Brain **Spinal cord**

Number of new cases annually: **16,000**

Number of deaths annually: **11,000**

Tumors of the brain and nervous system are uncommon. These cancers fall into many categories and are of variable malignancy.

Causes and risk factors
The causes of, and risk factors for, brain and nervous system tumors are unknown.

Types and development
About one third of brain and central nervous system tumors are secondary tumors (metastases) that have spread from primary tumors in other parts of the body. The other two thirds are primary tumors arising from the substance of the brain or its coverings. Gliomas arise from the supporting cells of the nervous system; meningiomas arise from the outer membrane coverings; pituitary adenomas arise from the pituitary gland; hemangiomas arise from the blood vessels of the brain; and pinealomas arise from the pineal gland. In children, the most common primary brain tumor, called a medulloblastoma, arises from the brain's primitive neuron-forming cells.

Primary tumors in the brain and nervous system expand, but they do not form secondary cancers outside the nervous system.

Symptoms and signs

Brain tumors quickly lead to an increase in pressure inside the skull. The pressure and the tumor itself have a wide range of effects, including headache, sudden vomiting, double vision, loss of part of the field of vision, partial paralysis, loss of sensation, seizures, and personality changes.

Diagnosis

Doctors use imaging methods, such as CT scanning and MRI, to detect brain tumors.

Treatment

Treatment is almost always surgical, often followed by radiation therapy. Success depends on the tumor's location and accessibility and the degree to which it has infiltrated other structures. New treatment methods are being developed.

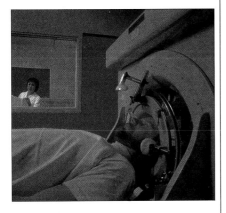

CT scanning
This man is lying with his head in a CT scanner, which rotates around the head and produces cross-sectional images that allow tumors to be detected.

Outlook

The prognosis varies with different tumors and with the safety with which the tumor can be removed. People with some gliomas have a 5-year survival rate of 50 percent; other gliomas are fast growing and may be fatal much sooner. People who have pituitary tumors or some types of meningiomas have 5-year survival rates of up to 90 percent.

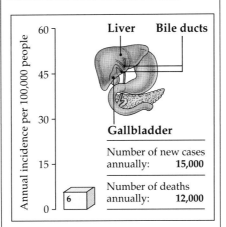

LIVER AND BILIARY TRACT CANCERS

Annual incidence per 100,000 people
Liver   Bile ducts
Gallbladder

| Number of new cases annually: | 15,000 |
| Number of deaths annually: | 12,000 |

Most liver cancers are secondary tumors that have resulted from the blood-borne spread of cancer cells from another part of the body, such as the breast, stomach, bowel, and lung. Primary liver and biliary tract cancers (including gallbladder cancers) are known as hepatobiliary cancers. Men are affected slightly more often by liver cancer, but cancer of the gallbladder is much more common in women. In general, blacks have a higher incidence of these cancers than whites. The highest incidence in the US is in Native Americans. Liver and biliary tract cancers occur most commonly in people over age 65. Primary liver cancer is more common in southeast Asia (including parts of China) and in tropical Africa, where it is the most common type of cancer in men.

Causes and risk factors

Hepatobiliary cancers occur most often when there is an existing disease. Cirrhosis and hepatitis B (and now hepatitis C) appear to predispose a person to primary liver cancer. Gallstones and parasites (such as liver flukes) are associated with gallbladder and biliary tract cancer. Alcohol abuse is a cause of cirrhosis, and therefore is linked with liver cancer.

Types and development

Most tumors begin in the cells of the liver or in the cells that line the gallbladder. Cholangiocarcinomas (cancers of the bile ducts) are rare and occur in conjunction with inflammatory bowel disease.

Symptoms and signs

The symptoms of hepatobiliary cancer include loss of weight and appetite, a feeling of discomfort in the upper right part of the abdomen, abdominal swelling, and sometimes a hard nodular mass that can be felt externally. Jaundice can also be a symptom. The symptoms are often not troublesome and in many cases no symptoms are noticed for weeks or months.

Diagnosis

Ultrasound, CT scanning, or MRI usually reveal the cancer. High levels of a substance called alpha-fetoprotein in the blood may indicate that the patient has a primary liver cancer.

Treatment

By the time most hepatobiliary cancers cause symptoms, they are not curable. If the tumor has not spread, surgery may be used to remove it. A transplant may be performed if the tumor has not spread extensively.

Outlook

Less than 5 percent of people with hepatobiliary cancer survive for 5 years after diagnosis.

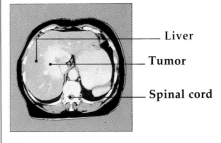

Liver
Tumor
Spinal cord

Liver cancer
This CT scan of a section of the abdomen shows a tumor of the liver.

LARYNGEAL CANCER

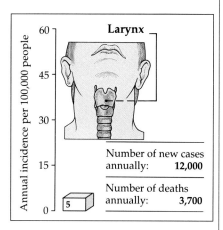

Larynx

Annual incidence per 100,000 people

Number of new cases
annually: **12,000**

Number of deaths
annually: **3,700**

Laryngeal cancer is becoming more common. Men are affected more often than women, and blacks more than whites. The peak incidence is at ages 60 to 75.

Causes and risk factors
Tobacco smoking is the major cause of laryngeal cancer; the incidence of laryngeal cancer in most countries parallels that of lung cancer. If a person stops smoking, the risk of laryngeal cancer begins to drop within 5 years after quitting and may reach the risk level of a lifelong nonsmoker after 10 years of not smoking.

Types and development
Most laryngeal cancers are of the squamous cell type. They may be supraglottic (above the vocal cords), glottic (on the cords), or subglottic (below the cords).

Symptoms and signs
The first symptom of laryngeal cancer is almost always a change in the voice, which may become hoarse or husky. Other symptoms include a sore throat, difficulty swallowing, or a mass that can be felt in the side of the neck.

Diagnosis
It is uncommon for primary care doctors to examine the vocal cords as part of a general physical examination unless there are already symptoms. However, any person who is at high risk (such as a person who has smoked heavily for many years) should ask his or her doctor to check the vocal cords for any premalignant changes or polyps. Diagnosis is by biopsy. CT scanning and MRI may help the doctor define the extent of the cancer's spread.

Treatment
Treatment depends on the extent of the disease, but usually includes surgery combined with radiation therapy. In cases that are discovered early, radiation therapy alone can preserve the vocal cords and thus the voice. In some cases of laryngeal cancer, treatment leaves the patient unable to speak. Other means of speaking can be devised, such as the use of an electronic voice enhancer adjacent to the trachea (windpipe).

Outlook
The 5-year survival rate varies from 60 to 80 percent, depending on the location of the cancer.

THYROID CANCER

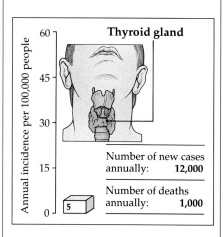

Thyroid gland

Annual incidence per 100,000 people

Number of new cases
annually: **12,000**

Number of deaths
annually: **1,000**

Thyroid cancer is uncommon. Its incidence has been increasing but seems to be stabilizing and is roughly the same throughout the world, except in Hawaii, Iceland, and Israel, where the rates are higher. Most people who have thyroid cancer are diagnosed between the ages of 25 and 65.

Causes and risk factors
Thyroid cancer affects twice as many women as men. The risk is increased when X-ray therapy is administered to adolescents for acne or other benign conditions.

Types and development
The main types of thyroid cancer are papillary adenocarcinoma, follicular carcinoma, and medullary carcinoma. Papillary and follicular carcinoma are the most common and are relatively slow growing; medullary carcinoma is much less common but is faster growing and metastasizes (spreads) early. Most thyroid cancers do not grow large enough to cause any symptoms; autopsies performed on people who have died of other causes show that about 6 percent have a cancer of the thyroid that caused no symptoms and so was never discovered.

Symptoms and signs
The first sign of thyroid cancer is a painless nodule in the neck, in or near the thyroid gland. Most thyroid nodules, however, are not cancers. There may also be airway obstruction and hoarseness if the tumor has grown large enough to produce a large goiter (thyroid enlargement).

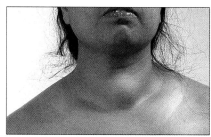

Thyroid cancer
The lump in this woman's neck is cancer of the thyroid gland.

Diagnosis

A thyroid scan may show that the glandular tissue in the nodule is either producing or is not producing thyroid hormone. This can help differentiate a benign tumor from a cancerous one. Definitive diagnosis is by biopsy.

Treatment

The main treatment for thyroid cancer is surgery, sometimes followed by radiation therapy or radioactive iodine treatment.

Outlook

The overall 5-year survival rate is between 90 and 95 percent. Recurrence is not uncommon.

MULTIPLE MYELOMA

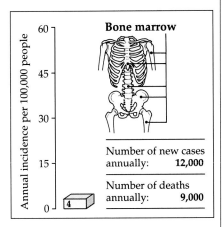

Bone marrow

Annual incidence per 100,000 people

Number of new cases annually: **12,000**

Number of deaths annually: **9,000**

Multiple myeloma is a cancer of the plasma cells – the cells of the body's immune system that produce antibodies. Multiple myeloma is slightly more common in males than females, and almost twice as common in blacks as whites. It rarely occurs before age 40; the highest rates occur in men over 80.

Causes and risk factors

Genetic factors may play a part, but exposure to certain chemicals is a likely cause, with increased rates in farmers and in workers exposed to heavy metals, asbestos, petrochemicals, and plastics.

Types and development

Plasma cell tumors most often develop in the bone marrow, often at several sites simultaneously, which is why this cancer is called multiple myeloma (myeloma means bone marrow tumor).

Symptoms and signs

A common symptom is back pain, caused by the tumor spreading to

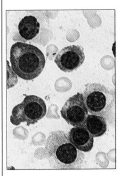

Multiple myeloma
This microscope picture of a bone marrow sample indicates multiple myeloma. It shows abnormal numbers of plasma cells (types of white blood cells).

the spine. Other symptoms or signs include anemia, abnormal bleeding, infections, and poor kidney function.

Diagnosis

A blood test may show an elevation of antibodies produced by plasma cells. X-rays of the back may show fractures or thinning of the bones. Definite diagnosis is made by biopsy of either the bone marrow or of one of the tumors.

Treatment

The main treatments for multiple myeloma are chemotherapy and radiation therapy. An alkylating drug can often bring about a complete remission, but just as often the disease returns. Radiation therapy is useful in helping to reduce the bone pain that affects most people with multiple myeloma. High-dose chemotherapy followed by bone marrow transplantation is being investigated.

Outlook

The overall 5-year survival rate is about 25 percent.

ESOPHAGEAL CANCER

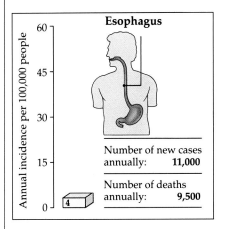

Esophagus

Annual incidence per 100,000 people

Number of new cases annually: **11,000**

Number of deaths annually: **9,500**

Esophageal cancer is an uncommon cancer, but one that usually has a poor outlook. It is more common in men than in women, and in blacks than in whites. It is most common in people between the ages of 55 and 65.

Causes and risk factors

Heavy use of alcohol and tobacco, particularly the use of the two together, increases the risk of esophageal cancer. Chronic inflammation and scarring of the esophagus are also risk factors. Nutritional factors may also play a part. Highly seasoned and spicy foods have also come under suspicion, though there has been little evidence to implicate them. Though inconclusive, a racial or genetic predisposition has been found in a few cases.

Types and development

The esophagus is a foot-long tube that carries food and fluids from the throat to the stomach. The majority of malignant tumors occur in the middle and lower parts of the esophagus. In some cases, cancer at the low end of the esophagus spreads down into the stomach and may cause obstruction; in other cases, the tumor is a stomach cancer that has spread up into the esophagus. Metastases, which occur in 50 percent of cases, are most common in the lymph glands.

Symptoms and signs
The most common symptoms are difficult or painful swallowing, loss of appetite, tiredness, and weight loss. There may also be noticeably swollen lymph glands or a hard mass that can be felt in the neck.

Diagnosis
Diagnosis can be made with a barium X-ray, or by direct inspection of the esophagus with a fiberoptic instrument. Biopsy of the tumor helps confirm the diagnosis.

Treatment
When possible, treatment includes surgery, which entails removal of a large part, or sometimes all, of the esophagus and any of the affected nearby tissues and lymph glands. The stomach, or sometimes a portion of colon, is pulled up into the chest during surgery and joined to the upper part of the esophagus to reestablish continuity of the gastrointestinal tract.

Outlook
The 5-year survival rate is about 5 percent.

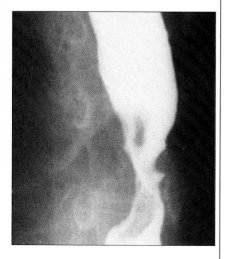

Esophageal cancer
This X-ray image of the esophagus shows a narrowed area, the result of blockage by a tumor.

TESTICULAR CANCER

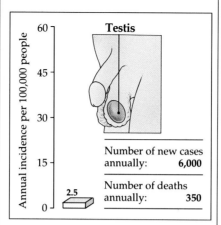

Testis

Annual incidence per 100,000 people

60

45

30

15

2.5

0

Number of new cases annually: **6,000**

Number of deaths annually: **350**

Testicular cancer is the most common cancer among men between the ages of 15 and 35, and the incidence is rising rapidly. The reasons for this trend are not clear. Whites are at four to five times the risk of blacks. Hispanics, Native Americans, and Orientals are at intermediate risk. There are significant geographical variations within the US, with the highest incidence in the San Francisco Bay area. Socioeconomic differences play a part, with the highest incidence among professionals. Testicular cancer is highly curable.

Causes and risk factors
Testicular cancer occurs most often in men who have had abnormal testicular development or who have had or still have an undescended testicle. The major risk factor for testicular cancer is an undescended testicle. The degree of risk is directly related to the degree of maldescent. Thus, a testis that is still in the abdomen has a one in 20 chance of becoming malignant, whereas if it is in the groin area it has a one in 80 chance of malignancy. The risk of testicular cancer is significantly reduced if the testicle is surgically brought down into the scrotum by age 8; the younger the patient is at the time of surgery, the less the risk.

Types and development
Testicular cancers are of two main types – seminomas (which involve the cells related to sperm production) and nonseminomas. The incidence of seminomas peaks in men in their 40s and 50s. Nonseminomas have a peak of incidence at about 20 years. Cancer may spread to the abdomen or lungs, the most common sites of metastases.

Symptoms and signs
Testicular cancer is symptomless in its early stages. The first sign is usually a painless bump on the surface of the testicle. Pain is a late symptom, by which time the cancer may have spread.

Diagnosis
Diagnosis is by the complete removal of the affected testis (orchiectomy). A biopsy is not done because testicular cancer is one of the few cancers in which biopsy can cause a spread of cancer cells.

Treatment
For a testicular cancer that has not spread, orchiectomy (performed as part of the diagnostic process) is also the main treatment. The other testis is also examined to ensure that it is free of cancer, which is usually the case. Depending on the kind of cancer and its severity, radiation therapy and/or chemotherapy may be used. Chemotherapy has dramatically improved the outlook for this cancer. The healthy testicle is shielded during radiation therapy. The removed testicle can be replaced with a prosthesis that looks and feels real. After treatment, most men have normal erectile function.

Outlook
The 5-year survival rate for men with testicular cancer is 90 percent, ranging from 50 percent for advanced cancers to nearly 100 percent for cases diagnosed early.

CONNECTIVE TISSUE AND OTHER SARCOMAS

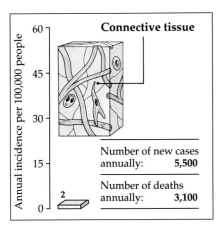

Connective tissue

Annual incidence per 100,000 people

60
45
30
15
0

| Number of new cases annually: | **5,500** |
| Number of deaths annually: | **3,100** |

Sarcomas are cancers of the bones, connective tissues, and other tissues, including the muscles, tendons, fibrous tissues, fat, blood vessels, and lining of the chest and abdominal cavities, and the coverings of the lungs, abdominal organs, and heart. All sarcomas of the connective tissues are rare. Males and females are affected equally, as are blacks and whites. Connective tissue cancers are more common in childhood and adolescence. One notable exception is Kaposi's sarcoma, a common complication of AIDS.

Causes and risk factors
The causes of most sarcomas are unknown. A few cases are pre-

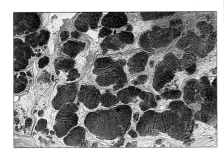

Sarcoma
In this microscope photograph, lung tissue (stained pink) has been invaded by a chondrosarcoma (purple), a cancer that has spread from the cartilage cells of bone.

sumed to be due to exposure to ionizing radiation, while others may be caused by intensive use of immunosuppressive drugs.

Types and development
Sarcomas can arise almost anywhere in the body, are very slow growing, and often recur locally after being removed.

Symptoms and signs
The most common symptom is a swelling that becomes progressively larger and more sore.

Diagnosis
Diagnosis is by a physical examination, X-ray, and biopsy.

Treatment
Treatment is by surgery, radiation therapy, and chemotherapy, depending on the type, grade, stage, and location of the cancer.

Outlook
In general, the outlook for people who have sarcomas can be good, with more than 50 percent of patients achieving long-term survival.

BONE CANCER

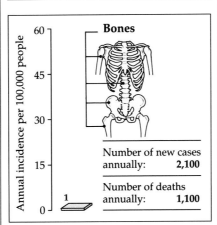

Bones

Annual incidence per 100,000 people

60
45
30
15
0

| Number of new cases annually: | **2,100** |
| Number of deaths annually: | **1,100** |

Cancers that originate in bone (primary cancers) are extremely rare. The incidence of primary bone cancer is the same worldwide, with blacks and whites and males and

females being affected at about the same rates. The peak age is in childhood and adolescence.

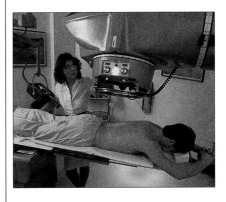

Treatment for spinal cancer
The photograph shows a man undergoing radiation treatment for spinal cancer. The light area on the patient's back is the target area for the radiation.

Causes and risk factors
There may be a familial predisposition to bone cancer, which is sometimes associated with genetic abnormalities or birth defects. Exposure to radiation is a risk factor. After 45, the cancer may occur with Paget's disease, a degenerative disease of the bone.

Types and development
Cancer can affect any bone, but typically affects the long bones (such as those in the arms or legs) in adolescence. There are two main primary bone tumors – called osteosarcoma and Ewing's sarcoma.

Symptoms and signs
Swelling over a bone that becomes progressively larger and tender may signal a bone cancer.

Diagnosis
Diagnosis is by X-ray of the area in question and by biopsy.

Treatment
Bone cancers are treated by surgery, radiation therapy, and chemotherapy, which has improved the outlook for these cancers.

Advances in surgery and bone transplantation can preserve the limbs.

Outlook

The addition of chemotherapy to radiation therapy and surgery has increased the 5-year survival rate to 55 to 80 percent.

EYE CANCER

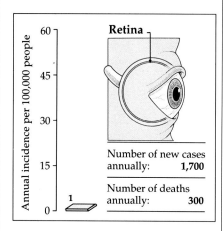

Cancer of the eye is a rare cancer that occurs in several different forms. It is equally common in males and females. One form (retinoblastoma) particularly affects children under the age of 5.

Causes and risk factors

Retinoblastoma results from a genetic abnormality. It arises from the outer layer of the retina.

Types and development

Retinoblastoma is a malignant tumor of the retina. It affects one or both eyes and is usually slow growing. Malignant melanoma, the most common eye tumor in adults, is also a slow-growing cancer. It is most common in the middle-aged and elderly and typically spreads to the liver.

Symptoms and signs

Squinting by a young child may be a sign of retinoblastoma. If the tumor is not detected in its early stages, it may be seen by a doctor as a white or yellow mass behind the pupil. Malignant melanoma often has no early symptoms, but it eventually causes a detached retina and distorted vision.

Diagnosis

Diagnosis is by examination of the eye using an ophthalmoscope (a viewing instrument). This is followed by CT scanning or MRI to assess the extent of the tumor.

Treatment

Small retinoblastomas can sometimes be treated by radiation therapy or laser treatment. However, the eye may eventually have to be removed to prevent spread of the tumor to the brain or elsewhere. When retinoblastoma occurs in both eyes, the eye with the larger tumor may be removed, and an attempt may be made to treat the other eye with laser therapy. In cases of malignant melanoma, the eye is removed when the tumor is discovered. It is not uncommon for the cancer to recur in the liver .

Outlook

The outlook depends on how far the tumor has spread before it is diagnosed and removed.

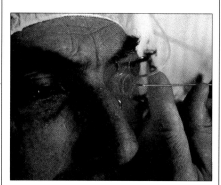

**Experimental treatment
for eye cancer**
A malignant melanoma of the eye is being treated here by experimental use of a laser, which activates an anticancer drug that has been introduced into the tumor.

VAGINAL CANCER

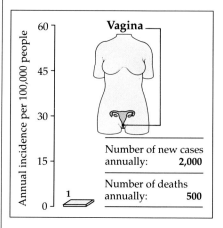

Cancer of the vagina is a rare cancer and the incidence appears to be decreasing.

Causes and risk factors

Increasing age is a risk factor, with most cases occurring in women between the ages of 50 and 70. The exact cause is not known, but radiation therapy has been implicated in about one fifth of the cases. It is thought that a history of uterine and vaginal prolapse, especially with prolonged use of a pessary to hold up a prolapsed uterus, is a risk factor.

Between 1940 and 1970, millions of pregnant women in the US who were spotting were given a synthetic estrogen called diethylstilbesterol (DES) to prevent miscarriage. It later was discovered that a type of vaginal cancer called clear cell adenocarcinoma was developing in the daughters of the women who took DES. The cancer occurred with greater frequency if their mothers had been given diethylstilbesterol before the fifth month of pregnancy.

Types and development

Squamous cell carcinoma accounts for more than 90 percent of vaginal cancers. Malignant melanoma and sarcoma occur infrequently. Clear cell adenocarcinoma is rare.

Symptoms and signs
There may be no symptoms until the cancer has grown or spread. Symptoms may then include bleeding or other discharge and painful sexual intercourse. Vaginal examinations and Pap smears may detect the cancer.

Diagnosis
Diagnosis is by biopsy.

Treatment
Depending upon its stage, vaginal cancer is usually treated by cutting out the cancerous tissue. Surgery with radiation therapy or radiation therapy alone may also be used.

Outlook
The 5-year survival rate is between 25 and 90 percent.

VULVAR CANCER

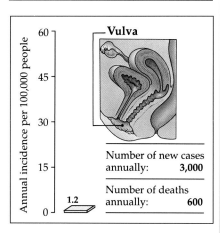

The vulva is the soft, skin-covered area surrounding the vaginal opening. The average age for acquiring vulvar cancer is 50 years.

Causes and risk factors
The exact cause of vulvar cancer is not known. It is more common in women who have diabetes and in women who are obese or who have high blood pressure, though the reasons for this are not clear. Venereal diseases have also been implicated as a cause of vulvar cancer.

Types and development
Almost all cases of vulvar cancer are of the squamous cell type, though there are some melanomas. Because the vulva is covered by skin, vulvar cancers are similar to squamous cell skin cancers, which can occur anywhere else on the surface of the body. The labia and clitoris are the most common sites of cancer of the vulva.

Symptoms and signs
The most common symptom of vulvar cancer is itching. Sometimes the affected person may feel a swelling. Other symptoms include pain (particularly during urination) and bleeding.

Diagnosis
Diagnosis is by biopsy.

Treatment
Surgery is the main treatment. Radiation therapy is also used. Anticancer drugs may also be applied directly to the cancer.

Outlook
Depending upon its stage, the overall 5-year survival rate is between 10 and 70 percent.

PENILE CANCER

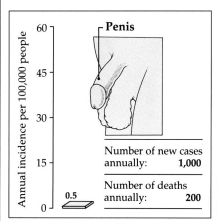

Penile cancer is more common in men from lower socioeconomic groups and in men who do not practice good hygiene. Penile cancer is rare in men under 25. The incidence in blacks is twice that in whites. The highest incidences in the world occur in Brazil and Africa, where the incidence is about 10 times that in the US.

Causes and risk factors
Poor hygiene has been associated with penile cancer. It has been suggested that the substance that accumulates under the foreskin of uncircumcised men, known as smegma, may be carcinogenic – a theory that is supported by the observation that penile cancer rarely develops in circumcised men (if circumcised as infants). It has also been suggested that the human papillomavirus (the wart virus) may cause cancer of the penis. Evidence of human papillomavirus infection has been found in some women with cervical cancer and subsequently in some men with penile cancer.

Types and development
Most penile cancers are of the squamous cell type, which develops into a crusting sore, usually on the head of the penis.

Symptoms and signs
More than half the men in whom symptoms develop delay seeking medical advice for more than a year after first noticing the symptoms. By this time, the lymph glands in the groin are often infiltrated with cancer and the chances of survival have been considerably reduced.

Treatment
Treatment is by radiation therapy and surgery to remove part or all of the penis. Any affected lymph glands are also treated.

Outlook
The 5-year survival rate is about 50 percent. Plastic surgery can be used to restore the penis.

INDEX

Page numbers in *italics* refer to illustrations and captions.

Photograph sources:
Biophoto Associates 83 (bottom)
Bubbles 61
The Image Bank 9; 48 (center); 49 (top right);
49 (bottom right); 55 (top right); 89;
98; 113; 120
Impact Photos 50 (top)
KeyMed 77 (bottom)
Living Technology 83 (center)
National Medical Slide Bank, UK 22; 44
(top center); 45 (bottom left); 49
(center right); 58 (bottom); 59 (top);
59 (center); 70 (bottom right); 71
(top); 71 (bottom); 84 (top right); 95
(inset); 109 (right); 128 (bottom); 129
(bottom); 134 (bottom); 136 (bottom
right); 137 (center)
Pictor International 40
Rex Features 52 (bottom left); 55
(bottom left)
Dr Norbert Roosen 98 (top inset); 98
(bottom inset)
Seidel Medizin 117 (top left)
Siemens 52 (bottom right)
Frank Spooner 54 (bottom)
Tony Stone Worldwide 114; 117
(top left)
Dr Paul Sweny 85 (bottom left)
The Telegraph Colour Library 19

John Watney Photo Library 133
(bottom)
Dr Ian Williams 70 (top right)
Dr Jennifer A. Young 80 (bottom)
Science Photo Library 2 (top left); 2 (bottom left); 2 (bottom right); 7; 14 (top);
14 (bottom left); 14 (bottom right); 26
(top left); 26 (bottom left); 26 (bottom
right); 27; 30 (top); 30 (bottom); 31
(left); 31 (right); 32 (center); 35; 36
(bottom); 44 (top right); 44 (bottom
left); 44 (bottom right); 45 (top left); 45
(bottom right); 48 (left); 50 (bottom);
55 (center right); 55 (bottom right); 57
(bottom left); 65; 70 (center right); 76
(top right); 76 (bottom right); 77 (top);
78 (bottom); 79 (top right); 79 (center
right); 83 (top); 84 (top left); 84 (center
left); 84 (bottom left); 84 (center right);
84 (bottom right); 85 (top); 85 (center);
85 (bottom right); 86 (bottom); 90; 91
(bottom); 96 (bottom); 105 (top); 108;
117 (top right); 118 (right); 121 (bottom
left); 122 (bottom); 123 (left); 124
(bottom); 125 (bottom); 126 (bottom);
127 (bottom); 130 (center); 130 (bottom); 132 (left); 132 (right); 135 (left);
135 (right); 138 (bottom); 139 (bottom
left); 139 (top right); 140 (bottom)

Front cover photograph:
© Lifestyle Productions International
1990/Telephoto

Commissioned
photography:
Steve Bartholomew
Susanna Price
Clive Streeter

Airbrushing:
Janos Marffy
Retouching:
Roy Flooks

Illustrators:
Russell Barnet
Karen Cochrane
David Fathers
Tony Graham
Andrew Green
Gilly Newman
Howard Pemberton
Lydia Umney
John Woodcock

Index:
Susan Bosanko

Reader's Digest Fund for the Blind is
publisher of the Large-Type Edition of
Reader's Digest. For subscription information about this magazine, please
contact Reader's Digest Fund for the
Blind, Inc., Dept. 250, Pleasantville, N.Y.
10570.